HARD TO STOMACH

REAL SOLUTIONS TO
YOUR DIGESTIVE PROBLEMS

JOHN MCKENNA

Newleaf

Newleaf
an imprint of
Gill & Macmillan
Hume Avenue, Park West
Dublin 12
www.gillmacmillanbooks.ie
© John McKenna 2002
978 07171 3369 7

Illustrations by Peter Bull Art Studio
Index compiled by Cover To Cover
Print origination by Carole Lynch, Dublin
Printed in Malaysia

This book is typeset in 11/14 Sabon.

The paper used in this book comes from the wood pulp of managed forests. For every tree felled, at least one tree is planted, thereby renewing natural resources.

A CIP catalogue record for this book is available
from the British Library.

15 16 17 18

CONTENTS

This book is dedicated to my son David. I love you very much and hope that we are not separated for much longer. I am proud of you because not only do you have such a kind heart but also great courage to deal with this separation.

CONTACT DETAILS FOR DR JOHN MCKENNA

Dr John McKenna
Nutrition Research Institute
15 Jigginstown Green
Naas
Co. Kildare
Tel: 045 897012
Email: nrinstitute@eircom.net

FOREWORD

This is a very important book in which John McKenna shares with his readers both his considerable knowledge and the successes that he has had in his practice of dealing with problems relating to digestion and stomach disorders, some of which may result in incurable illnesses.

Trained in orthodox medicine but with a wide knowledge in the field of complementary medicine, his research and practice has led to a clear understanding of how to deal with digestive problems effectively. As a result of his experience, he has drawn up programmes based on both orthodox and alternative treatments that actually work.

Both John and I realise ever more clearly, and over many years of practice, that the emphasis must be put on preventative medicine. Prevention is better than cure.

Conventional medicine teaches us how to overcome symptoms, but it is much more important that we look for the cause of illness in order to continue the treatment and find the cure for the source. Very little benefit is obtained by clearing up an ache or condition if we are not able to eliminate the cause. In order to do this we need to study the whole person and recognise what factors have contributed to each condition. There is usually a variety of reasons — for example, a breathing difficulty, a shortage of oxygen, a lack of rest or sleep. There are also many biological imbalances.

Over the years, and with great perseverance, John has developed an overall vision of total health that encompasses both the physical and mental circumstances of his patients. I am delighted that he is sharing his knowledge and experiences with us. He writes in a language that everyone can understand. I am very happy to recommend this book which will be of such relevance to so many people.

Dr h.c. Jan de Vries
Troon, Scotland

PREFACE

This book was inspired by the patients that I have treated over the last fifteen years in Ireland and in Africa. As with my book *Alternatives to Antibiotics*, I have found the need to express what I have observed from treating people. Digestive problems are unquestionably one of the commonest medical conditions world-wide. This book was written to help you, the reader, to identify when you or your loved one has a digestive problem and understand how to treat it. I have tried to write it as simply as possible with the minimum of jargon and the minimum of detail so as not to get bogged down. In this way I hope it is light, easy to read, humorous in places and informative. It draws mostly on my experience from treating hundreds of patients with digestive problems and I have included many case histories to illustrate certain points that I wanted to make.

There is a tremendous ignorance about food, nutritional supplements and what constitutes proper digestion. It amazes me on a daily basis how little people actually know. There is a great need for a nutritional awareness programme on television, radio, in schools, in clinics and at places of work. The more aware the general public becomes, the more society as a whole will benefit. The place to start an educational awareness programme is really with children when they are still quite young. They in turn will help to educate us adults and ultimately change the whole nature of society, creating a demand for healthier and safer food from the agricultural industry and others.

There also needs to be much more awareness about the role that digestion plays in our overall health. We need to become aware that we are a nation of chronically fatigued people, many of whom have mental and emotional problems such as irritability, anxiety and depression as a consequence of taking drugs such as antibiotics or the contraceptive pill or anti-inflammatories. The physical body interacts with and profoundly affects our mental and emotional well-being.

Most importantly, however, many people do not recognise that they have a digestive problem at all. The digestive system can be extremely silent even when there is serious pathology present. All too often patients come to a doctor for help when it is too late. I hope that I have emphasised in this book the importance of having your digestive system checked out by a practitioner of natural medicine to ensure that you are digesting and absorbing food correctly. I cannot emphasise this enough; many conventional doctors will do a colonoscopy at your annual check-up, or maybe only a blood test — this is not sufficient. Combine both natural and conventional forms of medicine to your own advantage and have a yearly check-up. Too many people take their digestive system for granted. Become aware and ensure that your body is nourished in an optimal way to ensure a long and healthy life; be aware and you will achieve your maximal potential as a human being.

I hope you learn something from reading this book and that it improves your health in a significant way.

John McKenna
March 2002

ACKNOWLEDGMENTS

Firstly, I would like to thank Eveleen Coyle of Gill & Macmillan for agreeing to publish this book and for being so supportive and helpful, not just during the publication of this book but also over the course of the last six years. Thank you Eveleen. Your belief in me has spurred me on to greater things.

I would also like to say a special thank you to my daughter Marianne for all her help with typing; her ability to spell medical terminology amazes me. She must have swallowed a medical dictionary when I wasn't looking. Thank you Nonny! I would also like to say thank you to my daughters Jackie and Charity for their love and support, especially during the last six years, which have been particularly challenging for all of us.

My sister Pauline and her husband Enda have been extremely kind to me throughout my life, but most especially over the last year. Your love and kindness mean a lot to me. Thank you.

Thanks also to all my patients in Capetown who have been very kind and supportive over the last five years; you have taught me much.

I would also like to say a special thank you to Maria Ascencao for her extraordinary support during my stay in Capetown. I shall not forget everything you did. To Maureen, Jackie, Rachel, thank you for all the wonderful help and support and advice; I miss you all.

Lameez, you have been through much, like myself, and I would like to thank you for your friendship. You are a very gifted healer; I wish you well.

During the last five years there has been one person who gave me hope, who helped me believe in life again and in whose company I felt alive again. Thank you Renata. You are a beautiful person and I am privileged to have known you.

Last but by no means least are my patients in Ireland, whom I've treated and who have written to me over the years after the publication of my books. You are the source of my inspiration and the reason why I have written books in the first place. Ireland is the most special country on the planet and Irish people are magical. Thank you for all your love and support.

1

THE DIGESTIVE SYSTEM

Figure 1.1 *THE DIGESTIVE TRACT*

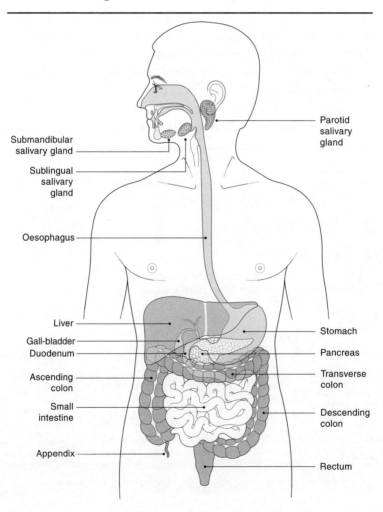

Digestion is really a very magical process in that we convert a piece of food, e.g. a potato, into tiny molecules (glucose) which will ultimately release energy in the cells of the body. It is the initial step in converting foodstuffs into energy.

The first step in this process of digestion involves breaking down large pieces of food into very tiny microscopic bits — so small that they will pass across the membrane of the cells lining the gut. This breakdown is done in two ways — physically and chemically. Physically we chew the food (at least we are supposed to). Our teeth help to tear and break up the food into smaller bits. Chemically, the food is broken down by means of enzymes, called digestive enzymes; this is the most important aspect of digestion.

To understand how enzymes function, let's look at how a protein is digested.

Figure 1.2 *THE DIGESTION OF A PROTEIN*

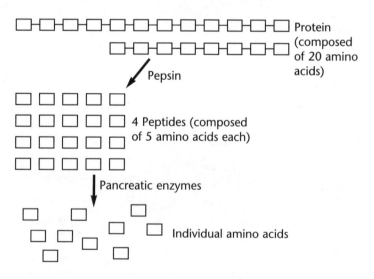

In the stomach, protein is mixed with digestive juices secreted by the cells lining the stomach. In these gastric juices there is an enzyme called pepsin. This chops large protein molecules into smaller, more manageable bits called peptides. The food then moves into the first part of the small intestine where the pancreas releases digestive juices, breaking the peptides down further to smaller peptides and then ultimately to amino acids. This is represented in Figure 1.2.

The same thing happens to carbohydrates (starch and complex sugars) and to fats and oils (lipids). They are all reduced to individual units, i.e. as simple a form as possible so that they can be transported across the gut wall into the bloodstream.

THE STAGES OF DIGESTION

THE MOUTH

Figure 1.3 *SALIVARY GLANDS*

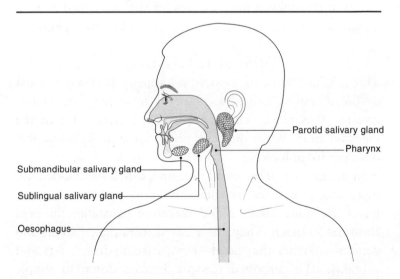

Years ago I did a training course in Austria called the Mayr Cure. We were given dry, hard bread rolls and were told to chew each bite fifty times before swallowing. After a few days of this you truly begin to learn the importance of chewing food. Prior to doing the course I used to gulp my food down as fast as possible and gave little heed to chewing.

In the mouth, food is chopped and torn down physically with the teeth. In addition, food is mixed with saliva, which is produced by the salivary glands (see Figure 1.3).

Saliva contains an enzyme called salivary amylase, which begins digesting starch. Food is chewed and mixed thoroughly with saliva before it passes down the oesophagus into the stomach.

STOMACH

The stomach produces gastric juices which are very acidic. Because acid can damage other parts of the digestive tract (the oesophagus above and the duodenum below), there are tightly controlled sphincters at either end of the stomach to prevent gastric juices from being released. The acid environment of the stomach kills off pathogenic bacteria and other harmful microbes; it also releases an enzyme called pepsin, which breaks down protein into smaller bits called peptides.

THE SMALL INTESTINE

This is where most of the action happens. It is where most of the digestion and absorption of food into the bloodstream takes place. Therefore, it is the critical bit of the digestive tract. When there are problems with digestion, this is where to go looking.

In the first bit of the small intestine, called the duodenum, more digestive juices are added to the food. These digestive juices are quite alkaline and therefore neutralise the acid from the stomach. They are released from the pancreas and contain enzymes that break down carbohydrates, fats and proteins. The carbohydrates are broken down to simple sugars (glucose, galactose), the protein is broken down to amino acids and the fats are broken down to fatty acids. However, since fat and water do not mix, the fat content of the diet must be emulsified with bile; in this way the fats and the digestive enzymes are brought into contact with one another to maximise digestion. People who do not produce sufficient bile cannot digest fatty foods and oils efficiently.

Further along the small intestine, more digestive juices are secreted by the wall of the small intestine. These complete the process of digestion by ensuring that any bits of food that were not fully broken down higher up in the gut are properly digested.

Once the food you eat has been reduced to molecule size it is then absorbed across the wall of the small intestine into the bloodstream.

ABSORPTION

Figure 1.4 *VILLI IN THE SMALL INTESTINE*

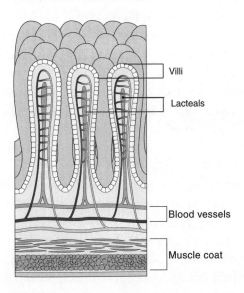

To make sure that most of the nutrients are absorbed, the wall of the small intestine is folded into villi — see Figure 1.4. When each villus is viewed under the microscope, it in turn is folded into millions of microvilli, increasing the surface area even more. This anatomical design ensures maximal surface area for absorption.

We have approximately five million villi, each about 1 mm long. They provide a surface area of roughly 10 square metres — about the floor area of an average bedroom.

The villi are filled with blood capillaries. When nutrients are absorbed into the bloodstream, they pass from the small intestine up to the liver. So the blood supply from the whole of the small intestine goes via the portal vein to the liver. This is an important fact to remember, because people with digestive problems can also end up with liver problems, and if the bowel becomes toxic, toxins will pass in the bloodstream to the liver, which can then come under a lot of strain — the liver is the main detoxifying organ in the body.

THE LARGE INTESTINE

Unabsorbed food and indigestible food such as roughage are moved along the small intestine and ultimately into the large intestine, or colon. In the large intestine water is re-absorbed, making the waste material, or faeces, more solid. If it is expelled too quickly from the large intestine, it will be excreted as diarrhoea; if it is held too long in the large intestine it will become very hard and lumpy.

The movement of faeces through the colon is made easier if it is filled with lots of roughage (i.e. fibre). When the rectum at the end of the large intestine becomes full, you get the sensation of wanting to pass a bowel motion.

In summary then, the digestive tract has three main functions: to digest, to absorb and to eliminate. Digestion occurs in the mouth, stomach and small intestine. Absorption of nutrients occurs mainly in the small intestine. Elimination occurs via the large intestine.

OTHER ORGANS CONNECTED TO THE DIGESTIVE SYSTEM

THE LIVER

The liver contributes bile to the process of digestion and is therefore regarded as a digestive organ. Bile, which helps to digest fats, is passed from the liver down the biliary tract and is stored in a little pouch called the gall-bladder. When you eat any foods containing fat (e.g. cream), the gall-bladder contracts and bile flows down the bile duct into the duodenum. Here bile emulsifies the fat globules in the food, allowing digestive enzymes to go to work and break down the fat globules to smaller units.

THE PANCREAS

The pancreas is also attached to the duodenum. It produces most of the digestive enzymes in the gastro-intestinal tract and is therefore the single most important organ associated with digestion. If this organ becomes stressed or damaged by viruses or vaccines or alcohol (or by gall-stones blocking the pancreatic duct), digestion becomes seriously impaired. As a consequence, poorly digested or undigested food can remain in the gut, where it ferments and putrefies.

This is why anyone with a digestive complaint should really assist the pancreas by taking a digestive enzyme supplement with each meal, as well as medicines to help heal the pancreas.

COMMON BOWEL PROBLEMS

DYSBIOSIS

Dysbiosis is unquestionably the commonest bowel problem, and has become especially prevalent in the last thirty years since drugs such as antibiotics, the pill, anti-inflammatories and steroids have become commonplace.

Dysbiosis means a disturbance in the bacterial population of the digestive tract. It occurs when some of the 'bad' bacteria increase in number as a result of some of the good bacteria being destroyed by drugs such as antibiotics, etc. (I shall discuss dysbiosis in detail in Chapter 3.)

PARASITES

Now that world-wide travel is much commoner, parasites are not a rarity anymore. Intestinal parasites should be suspected in anyone who complains of diarrhoea and a sore stomach. I test everyone who complains of digestive disturbances and I get a positive result in about 30 per cent of cases; in other words, one in three patients who come to see me (including children) with abdominal symptoms have intestinal parasites. This is an alarming percentage!

Parasites are hard to diagnose from a random stool sample, but fortunately detection methods have improved a lot over the last decade. Many laboratories suggest the use of an oral laxative to induce diarrhoea when testing for parasites, as this increases the level of detection. Some laboratories also suggest the use of a rectal swab, because some parasites live in the mucous membrane and so will seldom appear in stool; swabbing the area makes them easier to detect. It is always best to send samples to a laboratory that specialises in parasitology. Parascope Laboratories in Leeds, UK, is a university laboratory at the forefront of this field of medicine.

The commonest symptoms are:
1. Diarrhoea or irregular bowel motion
2. Abdominal bloating and discomfort
3. Lots of wind or flatulence
4. Loss of weight

If you suffer from two or more of these symptoms, ask your practitioner to check your stool sample for parasites.

FERMENTATION

Fermentation occurs when starches and sugars are not digested properly, and they 'go off' or ferment in the gut.

Fermentation requires an overgrowth of yeast, and therefore dysbiosis usually accompanies this condition, especially where *Candida albicans* and other species of candida have overgrown. This condition, therefore, should really be called fermentation dysbiosis but most practitioners refer to it simply as fermentation.

It produces symptoms such as fatigue, bloating and flatulence, especially after eating carbohydrates (sugars and starches), as well as a change in bowel habit. It causes the build-up of nasty chemicals that can enter the bloodstream and make the whole body toxic.

Treatment involves excluding all carbohydrates as well as excluding foods that could aggravate the dysbiosis — foods containing yeast and sugar as well as fermented products, malted foods and dried foods. As a result, it is a rather strict diet for the first few months. Treatment also involves the use of digestive supplements such as digestive enzymes. (I shall discuss this condition in more detail in Chapter 2.)

LEAKY GUT SYNDROME

The digestive system is a long tube, the lining of which is only one cell thick; this lining is called the mucosal barrier. This barrier blocks the entry of foreign substances into the bloodstream. If the mucosal barrier becomes inflamed or damaged, it can become leaky. Hence the term 'leaky gut syndrome'.

A healthy intestinal lining allows only completely digested food to pass across into the bloodstream; it also functions as a barrier to keep out bacteria, foreign substances and partly digested foods.

Figure 1.5 shows this mucosal barrier and shows how tightly packed the cells are.

There is a tight junction between adjacent cells which constitutes this barrier. However, when the lining becomes infected or inflamed this barrier becomes loose, allowing large molecules to pass through — undigested or partly digested food, bacteria, fungi and toxic chemicals from food or formed by gut fermentation. When these foreign substances enter the bloodstream they can trigger an immune response.

Figure 1.5 *TIGHT JUNCTIONS OR DESMOSOMES*

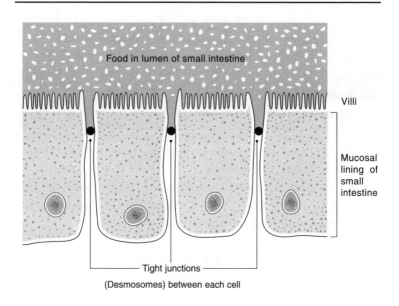

Leaky gut syndrome is associated with a range of medical problems, including food allergies, coeliac disease and Crohn's disease. It is also linked to a number of auto-immune diseases: asthma, atopy, eczema, ankylosing spondylitis, psoriasis, Reiter's syndrome and rheumatoid arthritis. Interestingly, childhood autism is strongly associated with leaky gut syndrome; autistic children develop significant reactions to gluten (found in wheat, rye, oats and barley) and casein (found in milk). Autistic children seem to react to the MMR vaccine with inflammation in the gut lining; it is this inflammation that causes the leaky gut, which allows proteins such as gluten and casein access to the bloodstream.

FOOD INTOLERANCES

'Doctor, ten years ago I was able to eat everything; five years ago I got indigestion and wind with wheat and dairy; two years ago I began to develop a reaction to other foods, restricting my diet even further. As time goes on I can eat less and less.'

This is something I have heard frequently over the years. It implies that the digestive process is impaired and is getting into more and more difficulty with time. When you react to a food, we say you suffer from a food intolerance. Lactose intolerance (lactose is the sugar found in milk) is the most common food allergy, although people can react to almost any food item. The foods that people react to most commonly include wheat, rye, dairy products, eggs, soya, citrus fruits, sugar and yeast. The foods that people almost never react to are rice and lamb.

Food allergies do not occur out of the blue for no good reason; there is usually an underlying digestive disturbance such as fermentation or leaky gut syndrome.

CASE HISTORY — BELINDA: FOOD ALLERGIES

Belinda was a high-powered lawyer who worked on a team for an international consulting firm. She often had to travel across the world and seldom had time to rest. While on a visit to London she developed a severe reaction to something in her evening meal and had to be admitted to hospital with anaphylactic shock — she became breathless as her airway started to close and she then went into a state of shock, which can happen if one develops a severe allergic reaction to something in the environment. All the medical tests that had been done in London indicated a food allergy, but they could not determine which food she had reacted to. She was very scared afterwards as she knew she could potentially go into shock anywhere at any time.

I was suspicious that there was an underlying digestive problem, and through a series of tests I discovered that the most likely diagnosis was leaky gut syndrome. The gut was inflamed and was not preventing certain substances from crossing the gut wall.

When proteins or peptides (partly digested proteins) enter the bloodstream, there is an immediate allergic response, since neither protein nor peptides should be in the bloodstream; they have to be broken down into amino acids before being allowed into the bloodstream. In people with leaky gut syndrome, undigested food substances can leak directly from the gut into the bloodstream and can cause the kind of severe reaction that Belinda had.

It was necessary to use a strict diet for a period of six months, which allowed the digestive tract to heal. In addition, I used probiotics, glutamine and a number of digestive supplements. I also recommended that she change her job, as it was not possible to follow the treatment regimen that I had proposed while travelling and following her hectic schedule. Her boss agreed to base her at head office for one year to facilitate treatment. I also recommended that she go for stress management. She made excellent progress and has left the corporate world and is now managing a small farm. She is able to digest many foods now which she was previously allergic to — clear testimony to the fact that the digestive system can heal; it does, however, take time.

Food intolerances or allergies are usually associated with digestive disturbances. These digestive disturbances include fermentation, dysbiosis, leaky gut syndrome and inadequate digestive enzymes.

Food allergies or intolerances are interesting in that the effects are often delayed. With a classic allergy, say to cats or pollen, the reaction is immediate; however, with reactions to food the effect can be delayed for hours. What is also very interesting is the fact that people with an allergy to a food such as wheat, for example, often crave that food. This can lead to bingeing on that same food.

Most reactions to food are not life-threatening and so do not require hospitalisation. But what about Belinda's case?

Medical immunologists now agree that it is possible, though not common, to develop a full-blown anaphylaxis to a food such as wheat. One allergy specialist, Dr Braly, Director of Immune Laboratories in the US, has seen a number of patients who show both an immediate as well as a delayed reaction to food.

The immediate type of reaction to allergies such as cats or pollen is called an IgE type reaction. IgE is a type of antibody that is found attached to mast cells, which can release histamine and other chemicals that cause the typical symptoms of an allergy — rhinitis, itchy skin, skin rash, wheeze, etc.

Delayed reactions, which include most food allergies, are not of the IgE type and so do not give the typical allergy symptoms. Food allergies seem to be IgG type reactions — IgG is another class of antibody. It is not found attached to mast cells and hence the absence of the typical allergy symptoms. This delayed food allergy, IgG type, appears to be a result of quantities of partially digested and undigested food entering the bloodstream. The immune system will detect this foreign protein and try to render it harmless by attaching IgG antibodies to it.

Figure 1.6 shows a list of symptoms associated with food allergies. If you have any of these symptoms, consult your practitioner and find out which foods you are allergic to.

Remember that the foods you crave are often the ones that you are allergic to.

WHICH FOODS CAUSE ALLERGIES?

Well, almost any food can but the most common are the following:

Wheat (bread, biscuits, flour, pasta)
Milk products (cheese, yoghurt, cream)
Eggs
Soya (soya milk, soya flour, tofu, miso)
Coffee
Tea
Chocolate
Nuts

Oranges

Chemical additives in food (MSG, tartrazine, etc.)

If you find that you 'cannot live' without one or more of these foods, it may be worth your while having allergy tests done.

Figure 1.6 *20 SYMPTOMS SUGGESTIVE OF A FOOD ALLERGY*

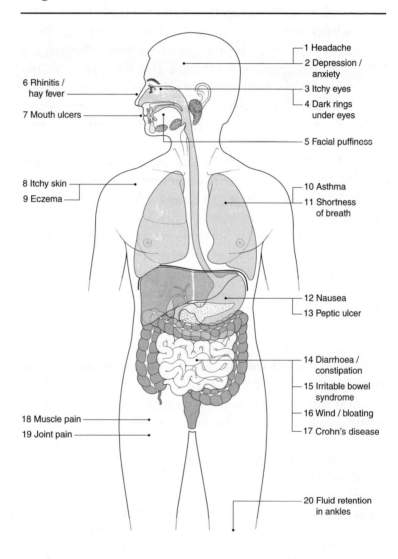

CAUSES OF DIGESTIVE DISTURBANCES

So far we have looked at some of the digestive problems that people suffer from. Now let's examine the causes of these problems. Top of the list must come stress.

STRESS

When you are actually stressed (e.g. before an exam), you get butterflies in your tummy, nausea and occasionally vomiting (I've seen a few footballers get sick before an important match during my footballing days). In other words, your digestion gets disturbed. If the stress goes on and on day after day, i.e. becomes chronic, you end up having difficulty digesting the food you eat. Also, when you are stressed you tend to eat faster and chew less and do not rest after eating.

The French take three hours off in the middle of the day to have lunch and yet they do well economically. They have excellent eating habits and have a great knowledge not only of nutrients but also of the process of digestion. For example, before eating they will use an aperitif, which contains bitter substances that stimulate the production of digestive juices, thereby preparing the digestive system for food. The alcohol content of the aperitif calms you down as does wine with a meal.

One of the golden rules is to never eat when stressed or anxious. Rather use a natural relaxant such as Kava Kava (for further details see my book *Alternatives to Tranquillisers*). Many people with digestive problems will not tolerate alcohol well, so try to avoid wine and beer and any other alcoholic drink.

Stress is a major factor in irritable bowel syndrome, in gut fermentation, in pancreatic insufficiency (not enough digestive enzymes being produced) and in dysbiosis. Belinda was a good example of someone who was very stressed at work and did not want to accept it. It was only when she developed a life-threatening food reaction that she came to her senses. I shall discuss stress and its effects on digestion in more detail in Chapter 4.

DRUGS

The second major cause of digestive problems is conventional, medical drugs. These include antibiotics, steroids, anti-inflammatories, such as brufen, ponstan etc., and the contraceptive pill.

ANTIBIOTICS

Treatment with any antibiotic for an infection and the long-term use of antibiotics in the treatment of acne is liable to alter the balance of the intestinal flora; very strong antibiotics such as clindamycin and lincomycin may cause drastic changes. Oral antibiotics often cause gastro-intestinal disturbances, especially in young children. Many complain of vague symptoms such as nausea, a dull ache in the tummy and a sickly feeling all over the abdomen. Others have more definite symptoms such as diarrhoea — probably the commonest side-effect of antibiotic therapy — flatulence, bloating and loss of appetite. Long-term problems can range from allergies and recurrent infections to more serious problems such as dysbiosis, diabetes and liver damage.

Because of the increased susceptibility to illness after antibiotic therapy, it is very important to re-establish the intestinal flora as soon as possible. When on a course of antibiotics, take a supplement of 'good' bacteria called a probiotic. Table 1.1 shows some of the adverse effects of antibiotics on the digestive tract. If I see any of these effects in a patient, I will immediately test the bacterial population to see if it is disturbed and treat it if it is (see Chapter 3 for treatment).

Table 1.1 *ADVERSE EFFECTS OF ANTIBIOTICS*

Effects on the digestive tract
  abdominal pain/discomfort
  sickly feeling in the stomach
  increased flatulence (wind)
  alteration to bacterial flora
  pancreatic damage

Nutritional effects
  a decrease in the level of certain minerals (zinc, calcium, magnesium)
  a decease in the level of certain vitamins (K, B_2, B_3)

General effects
  tiredness
  altered mood
  impaired immune response

THE CONTRACEPTIVE PILL

The oestrogen component of the pill is known to alter the bacterial flora and so can cause digestive complaints; not everyone who takes the pill gets digestive complaints but most do.

Abdominal bloating, changes in bowel habit, headache, tiredness, vaginal thrush and mood swings are the commonest complaints associated with the contraceptive pill.

If a woman is using the pill as the sole means of contraceptive, it is often hard to convince her to come off it while the digestive system is being treated, though this is especially important if she has dysbiosis (abnormal bacterial population). It is very difficult to treat dysbiosis effectively if someone insists on using the pill, as it is a drug that is known in conventional medicine to disturb the bacterial population of the digestive tract. So if you have been on the pill, have a stool analysis done.

ANTI-INFLAMMATORY DRUGS (NSAIDs)

These drugs are used to treat fever and inflammatory conditions such as arthritis, trauma, etc., and are also used as painkillers. They are commonly used in sports injuries and in the treatment of all forms of arthritis to relieve pain and inflammation. In pharmacy, this class of drugs is called non-steroidal anti-inflammatory drugs, which is abbreviated to NSAIDs. Examples of NSAIDs include brufen, ponstan, voltaren and ibuprofen.

All NSAIDs damage the lining of the digestive tract and should be used with great caution in someone who already has a digestive problem. My sister, for example, had a duodenal ulcer and was put on one of these drugs for pain relief. She ended up in hospital with a bleeding ulcer.

NSAIDs damage not only the digestive tract but the kidneys as well, so be careful. I am shocked to see such drugs being used to treat fever in small children.

By damaging the lining of the gut, they alter the whole ecology of the gut, and this can take a long time to repair. Many people who use them on an ongoing basis for arthritis end up with very significant gastro-intestinal problems, such as dysbiosis, fermentation and leaky gut syndrome.

If you have used these drugs and have suffered or are presently suffering from a digestive disturbance, seek treatment from a practitioner.

STEROIDS

Steroids produce side-effects in every system of the body. They disturb the hormonal system and therefore the whole body chemistry. A short course of less than seven days will not produce much in the way of side-effects, but repeated courses, and when used for longer periods of time, especially for more than two weeks, can result in significant side-effects.

Steroids produce similar side-effects to the NSAIDs in the digestive tract and are implicated in a range of bowel disorders from dysbiosis to fermentation.

If you have been on steroids, have your digestive system checked out by someone with experience in this field. Generally naturopaths, homeopaths and acupuncturists are all well trained and are aware of the damage that these drugs can inflict on the digestive tract.

INVESTIGATING THE DIGESTIVE TRACT

I am going to contrast the ways in which conventional and alternative medicine investigate the digestive system. This will help explain why GPs and specialists, after having done a series of tests, will say that there is nothing wrong, despite the fact that you are suffering significant symptoms. Firstly, let's see how conventional medicine sets about investigating the digestive system.

Conventional medicine tends to be very invasive, sticking tubes in, sticking probes or needles in, invading the body's cavities. Generally it is assumed that if a problem cannot be seen there is no problem. As a consequence, the most reliable investigation in conventional medicine involves passing a tube down the oesophagus into the stomach and through to the first part of the duodenum. This investigation is called a gastroscopy. The tube is called an endoscope and it enables the doctor to see the lining of the whole of the upper gut — oesophagus, stomach and duodenum. It shows up cancer, ulcers, inflammation, reflux and other problems.

An endoscope can also be used to see the bottom end of the digestive tract, i.e. the rectum and the whole of the colon. Here it is possible to diagnose cancer, diverticulitis, Crohn's disease, colitis and other conditions.

However, the most important part of the digestive system, the small intestine, lies beyond the range of both of these endoscopes and so cannot be visually investigated. The small intestine is the most important part of the digestive system because it is here that practically all of the digestion and all of the absorption take place. In other words, most of the important functions of the digestive system occur here. Conventional medicine seems to have no effective means of testing the small intestine.

Alternative medicine, on the other hand, investigates in a very different way, using saliva, stool and urine.

SALIVA

Practitioners of natural medicine often test the saliva first. This is to test the pH (acidity or alkalinity) of the saliva, which is a good indicator of the body's pH balance. Many people with digestive problems are very acidic and so have a low salivary pH. Salivary pH is tested using litmus paper. If the paper turns blue when mixed with saliva, it means that the person is too acidic and may well have a digestive problem. This is a very cheap and simple test that you can do at home.

Normal pH values for saliva are 6.2 to 6.4. If the pH is below 6.0 then it indicates too much acidity.

STOOL

Secondly, practitioners will test a stool sample for:
(a) bacterial flora
(b) microscopic parasites
(c) worms

URINE

Thirdly, the urine is sent to a laboratory for:
(a) biochemistry — pH, protein, sugar, ketones, etc.
(b) indican — a test to see how well you digest food.

In this way three major digestive disorders can be diagnosed — dysbiosis, fermentation and parasitic infestation. The bacterial flora test will show if there is dysbiosis and will quantify it, giving you an indication of how badly the flora is disturbed. Repeat tests after treatment will gauge progress in a scientific way. The stool analysis may also reveal the presence of parasites. By parasites I mean *micro*scopic single-celled animals, for example, *Entamoeba histolytica*, which cause amoebic dysentery; I do not mean worms. Worms are *macro*scopic and so can be seen with the naked eye. A good stool analysis should check for eggs, cysts and whole worms as well.

The urine test should test the biochemistry of the urine, i.e. check the pH (should be between 5.0 and 7.0), check for proteins, glucose, ketones and blood, all of which should be negative — ketones are present only if fasting or in diabetes.

A good biochemistry result would read as follows:

Urine pH — 6.0
Glucose — negative
Protein — negative
Ketones — negative
Blood — negative

The indican test indicates how well you are digesting food. If food is poorly digested, the carbohydrates will ferment and the proteins will putrefy and produce toxic chemicals such as indican, which will then appear in the urine. This is a very cheap test and is a quick and helpful way of gauging one's digestive ability. It is an old-fashioned test and so not every laboratory does it.

The urine can also be tested for other substances. For example, the best way to test for leaky gut syndrome is the mannitol and lactulose test; these are two sugars that we do not metabolise, so they will be excreted in the urine unchanged. Mannitol is readily absorbed across the gut wall because it is a small molecule; lactulose is poorly absorbed because it is a much larger molecule. Therefore, if you are absorbing food correctly, the urine will show high levels of mannitol and very low levels of lactulose; if there are high levels of both mannitol and lactulose then it indicates leaky gut syndrome — large molecules are leaking across the gut wall into the bloodstream and then excreted in the urine.

All in all, alternative medicine is much less invasive and

uses saliva, stool and urine to diagnose what is happening inside the digestive tract. Alternative medicine also tests the most important part of the digestive tract, the small intestine, via stool and urine tests. It is in the small intestine that we find leaky gut syndrome, some parasites such as *Giardia lamblia*, most worms, and it is also where we go looking for fermentation problems.

INVESTIGATING THE DIGESTIVE SYSTEM

Table 1.2 *CONVENTIONAL MEDICINE VS. ALTERNATIVE MEDICINE*

Conventional Medicine	Alternative Medicine
1. Invasive	1. Non-invasive
2. Uses a gastroscope or colonoscope	2. Uses stool, urine and saliva
3. Seldom tests for dysbiosis, fermentation, parasites	3. Commonly tests for dysbiosis, fermentation, parasites
4. Has difficulty detecting problems in small intestine	4. Can easily detect problems in the small intestine
5. Can test upper and lower parts of digestive system	5. Can test all parts of the digestive system.
6. Expensive	6. Inexpensive

Investigation of the small intestine is critical in diagnosing and treating digestive problems. The small intestine is the supply line for nourishment to the rest of the body. If it is in difficulty, the rest of the body will be in difficulty as well, hence the wide range of symptoms that digestive disorders can produce. If you look back at Figure 1.6, which shows how food allergies in the digestive tract can create such an array of symptoms, affecting many parts of the body, you'll see what I mean. Digestive disturbances not only affect one's physical well-being, but also one's mental, emotional and spiritual well-being, as you will learn throughout the remainder of this book.

SUMMARY

The anatomy of the digestive system is quite simple; it is a long tube, approximately 10 metres in length, with a lining that is one cell thick, called the mucosal barrier. However, its function is quite complex in that it has to digest food enzymatically, it has to allow the absorption of small molecules into the bloodstream while keeping bigger molecules out, and it has to eliminate wastes. It serves a critical role in one's immunity in that it is lined with billions of 'soldiers' ready to fight off any invaders; these are called the 'good' bacteria or the intestinal flora. It also has a brain in that all the structures that are found in the central nervous system — sensory cells, neurons, neurotransmitters and hormones — exist in the digestive system. As a result, one's emotions are often reflected in the digestive tract; for example, acute stress can lead to nausea and/or diarrhoea. Because digestion is adversely affected by stress and by conventional drugs, digestive disorders are very common in the modern world. The commonest disorders include dysbiosis, fermentation, leaky gut syndrome and food allergies or intolerances. In contrast to conventional medicine, natural medicine favours simple, inexpensive and non-invasive tests that involve collecting samples of saliva, urine and stool. Also in contrast to conventional medicine, natural medicine focuses a lot of effort on testing the most important part of the digestive tract, which is the small intestine; it is here that most of the digestion and absorption takes place and so it is here that most problems occur.

2

FERMENTATION IN THE GUT

Fermentation is a disorder of the small intestine (see Figure 2.1). It does not imply that there is a problem with elimination; rather it suggests a problem with digesting food efficiently. In other words, you can have a perfectly regular bowel motion once or twice a day but still have a very significant digestive disturbance. I have found that patients have often confused these two issues. When taking a medical history I ask if the patient has any digestive problems, only to be told that everything is normal in that department, as he/she has a bowel motion every morning like clockwork.

A normal bowel habit does not equate to a normal digestive system.

If you look at Figure 2.1, you will see that elimination of waste from the digestive system is a function of the large intestine or colon. When faeces enters the large intestine it is in a liquid state. The function of the large intestine is to remove water from it, thereby making it more solid.

Impairment of the functioning of the small intestine is far more serious than that of the large intestine. The small intestine is responsible for the digestion and absorption of food, both of which are critical for your overall health — the food you eat is broken down, absorbed and then used to nourish the rest of your body. As you can now appreciate, the small intestine is the most important part of the digestive tract; you cannot survive without it. By contrast, anyone can do without their large intestine and indeed some people have to, when it is removed surgically for such conditions as ulcerative colitis, Crohn's disease, cancer of the colon, etc.

Figure 2.1 *THE FUNCTION OF THE SMALL AND LARGE INTESTINES*

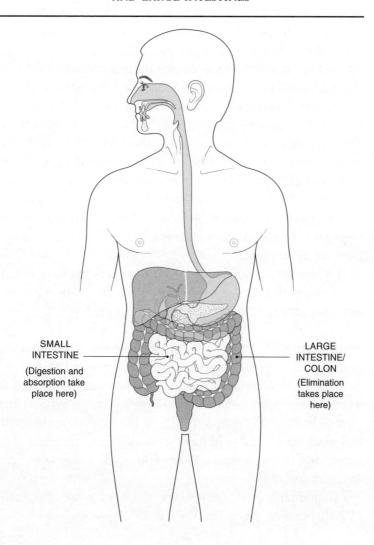

Impairment of the small intestine is a slow, insidious process and can go unnoticed even when well advanced. Unlike the skin, which is well supplied with nerves, the small intestine has a poor nerve supply and is therefore less able to warn you when things go wrong. This is why a problem like fermentation can develop without your being aware of it.

CASE HISTORY — JAN: CANCER OF THE PANCREAS

While I was doing my hospital training an elderly gentleman was admitted to the ward for investigation. He was complaining of vague discomfort in his abdomen as well as loss of appetite. He had lost ten kilograms in weight over the previous two months. All the intestinal investigations — barium meal, follow-through and colonoscopy — as well as numerous blood tests, were reasonably normal. He was then scheduled for an exploratory laparotomy, where the surgeon cuts open the abdomen to see the state of each organ. I assisted at the operation and as we opened the abdomen wall it was obvious that the whole abdominal cavity was riddled with cancer, which is what we had suspected. As the cancer was too far advanced it was not possible to remove it and so we just closed the abdomen again and sent him back to the oncology ward for assessment.

This case history will always stand out in my mind, as it illustrates well how a disease can be very advanced in the abdomen and still produce little in the way of acute symptoms.

Fermentation is a functional disorder of the small intestine and implies that digestion is impaired. I explain this to my patients by saying that if you leave some meat, potatoes and vegetables — a normal lunch or dinner — in a glass of water overnight and ask people to eat it the next day, they will refuse to do so as it will have gone off, i.e. fermented. *The starch and sugar content will ferment, while the protein content will putrefy.*

In summary then, fermentation occurs when the small intestine cannot digest food efficiently. It is a disorder of the small intestine and may have no effect on the bowel habit whatsoever.

How Does Fermentation Occur?

Fermentation is a rare disorder among the primitive peoples that I have lived with, e.g. the Fulani in West Africa or the San people of southern Africa. It is a disorder of Western civilisation. It has to do with our lifestyle and the food we eat and the way in which we eat it.

The single commonest cause of fermentation is stress. When you are acutely stressed (e.g. before an exam) you get butterflies in your tummy or your tummy gets very upset. You are aware that if you eat food at this time you may feel nauseous and may even vomit or have diarrhoea. The reason for this is that stress raises the level of adrenaline in the bloodstream, which shifts blood away from the digestive tract to the muscles in preparation for action. If the stress then becomes chronic, your ability to digest food may be significantly impaired. The stress may be external, e.g. pressure at work, or it may be internal, e.g. emotional upheavals. Considering the fact that many people are under increasing pressure these days, especially time pressure, and considering the fact that many people also have deep-seated emotional issues to deal with, it is not surprising that fermentation is not an uncommon disorder. Add to this our eating habits and the poor quality of many people's diets and it is a wonder that we are all still alive and semi-well.

The Foods We Eat and the Way We Eat Them

When I was at medical school there was always too much to do and not enough time to do it. As a consequence, meals were often a very hurried affair. Breakfast consisted of coffee and a bar of chocolate, lunch was a hot dog or hamburger and supper was often a takeaway pizza or Chinese meal. The sugar and starch content of my diet was way too high, with minimal fruit and vegetables. Too much starch can predispose you to fermentation, especially if you are also stressed at the same time. To treat fermentation, it is necessary to exclude starch and sugars from your diet, as both can ferment easily and produce alcohols in the gut, hence giving you that drunk or hungover feeling.

The quantity of food consumed can also predispose you to fermentation. We have been conditioned by our society to eat three square meals a day, regardless of whether or not we are actually hungry. We eat far too much and too often, considering the fact that many of us lead quite sedentary lives and exercise insufficiently. When we eat out at a restaurant, we feel obliged to finish everything on the plate, irrespective of whether we feel full or not. To overload the digestive tract with food puts stress on it and can impair the digestive process. There is a built-in feedback mcchanism in your body to tell you when you have had enough to eat, but you have to listen to it. Take time to eat, and eat smaller meals, because heavy meals can put a tremendous workload on your digestive capacity.

The way we eat is probably the most important predisposing factor of the lot. Many of us eat on the run while trying to do other things at the same time. When I attended medical school, eating was something to be completed as quickly as possible, as I had more important things to do. It was only when I did a training course on natural medicine in Austria many years later that I began to accept the importance of eating slowly and focusing your whole being on the process instead of reading a book or opening the mail or watching television, as I used to do. I now understand why the French take so long over lunch and allow time for the digestive enzymes to break down the food before resuming work. The course in Austria taught me the importance of eating slowly, never eating when stressed or tired, and never eating when reading the newspaper or watching television, as these activities can make you tense. The training course in Austria was a real eye-opener, but it supported what I had always believed, i.e. an efficient digestive tract is the key to good health.

Here are the rules for healthy eating:

1. Take time – do not rush. Leave at least one hour.
2. Chew the food well and mix it well with the saliva.
3. Be relaxed. Do not eat if stressed or tired; rather de-stress or rest.
4. Taste the food and savour every bite.
5. Do not be distracted with letters, newspapers, television, etc.
6. Eat the main meal in the middle of the day and little in the evening.

Symptoms of Fermentation

The symptoms associated with fermentation can be few or many, subtle or obvious; they can be either associated with the digestive system or associated more with other parts of the body. Let's look at the digestive symptoms first.

Fermentation can cause a host of digestive symptoms, but the most common are flatulence, which can be quite excessive, abdominal bloating, diarrhoea or constipation, active bowel sounds (gurgling sounds), early morning nausea. There may also be some degree of abdominal discomfort due to the flatulence. The tongue is often coated and the breath may have an unpleasant odour.

When fermentation persists untreated, the rest of the body begins to suffer and non-abdominal symptoms become prominent. These include low energy, loss of interest/motivation, mood swings, irritability, sleep disturbances, headaches, nasal congestion, cold hands and feet, exhaustion upon waking. There may also be increased sweating. These secondary symptoms are quite non-specific and many doctors fail to link them with digestive problems. Let us look at some of these symptoms in more detail. The following case histories clearly illustrate some of the main symptoms of fermentation.

CASE HISTORY — BARRY: EXCESSIVE BELCHING

A 42-year-old man came to see me complaining of excessive belching. He said that he was belching up to eighty times a day and that it was noticeably worse after eating. He found it very embarrassing as he had to deal with business clients every day and some of them had commented on his habit of belching. He had a very stressful job dealing with financial investments on the internet, and because he had become self-employed in the last two years he had to work very long hours and often at weekends as well. He had been to his GP, who had done various investigations on him, all of which were negative. The doctor told him to take a holiday and that would solve his problem. Because I've had fifteen years of dealing with similar cases to his, it was quite easy to diagnose his problem within a few minutes of speaking to him. Unfortunately not all patients are as easy to diagnose as Barry. On examining him his abdomen was distended and very resonant when I percussed with my fingers. On listening with the stethoscope the bowel sounds were excessively active. I then asked him to do a urine and stool test so that I could confirm the diagnosis. Two days later the results confirmed that he did indeed have intestinal fermentation. I then treated him with a gut fermentation control diet plus digestive enzymes and a herbal remedy to assist his digestive tract. I also added grapefruit seed extract as an anti-fungal agent, since fermentation is often associated with overgrowths of yeast in the wall of the intestine — you need yeast to ferment.

One month later there was a remarkable improvement in his condition. The belching was now minimal and associated with dietary indiscretions, especially after eating sugary foods. His energy was improved and he was sleeping better and was waking up refreshed rather than hungover. I then repeated the tests and confirmed the improvement. When he saw the improved results he felt good about himself and was encouraged to continue treat-ment. This involved broadening his diet to allow for a little carbohydrate and some more fruit, oats, rye and pulses. By the end of the second month the belching had stopped completely and he felt much stronger and healthier. He was also much better able to handle the stress at work and had decided to employ an assistant to enable him to spend more time with his family.

The production of excess gas in the digestive tract is a cardinal symptom of fermentation.

As anyone who does home-brewing will tell you, gas is a by-product of fermenting beer or wine; in the same way, the digestive tract will also produce lots of gas as a by-product of gut fermentation. The above case history illustrates this point very well.

The next time you see someone belching a lot you will be able to advise them what to do.

CASE HISTORY — KEVIN: HALITOSIS

Kevin was twenty-five years old and was suffering from bad breath, or halitosis. His family and girlfriend had told him to get help for it; hence his visit to me. He was a relaxed kind of guy but was under a lot of stress as he was trying to work and study at the same time and so he had little relaxation time in his day. He was a full-time student at university and he also had a part-time job as a waiter in a busy restaurant. Because of this hectic schedule he had an erratic eating pattern, snatching meals where he could. Much of what he ate consisted of starch — bread, pasta, potatoes, hamburgers and hot dogs, etc., and very little fruit and vegetables.

Kevin also complained of having a strong body odour on occasion, as well as very heavy sweating, especially at night. He often had to change his pyjamas in the middle of the night. His hands and feet were cold and clammy. On examining him he had a thick white coating on his tongue, his hands and feet were indeed cold and clammy and his abdomen was very tender, especially in the area around the umbilicus. His liver edge was acutely tender when I pressed under the right ribcage.

He had a nasty case of athlete's foot, which is a fungal infection of the skin between the toes and on the soles of the feet. His fingernails had numerous white spots, there was swelling of the skin around the base of his nails and the skin was peeling.

I did a urine and stool test to ascertain the cause of the halitosis and I also did a blood test to assess his liver function. Fortunately the latter was normal, but the urine test indicated that he had intestinal fermentation, and the stool test showed numerous pus cells as well as *Giardia lamblia* cysts and a significant overgrowth of *Candida albicans* in fungal form.

Because Kevin had a number of intestinal problems, it was no small wonder that he had bad breath, as his whole digestive tract was under great strain.

It is difficult to correct the bacterial flora of the intestine when there is a fermentation process going on at the same time, as you will learn shortly from another case history. Therefore I set about correcting the fermentation problem initially.

As in the case of Barry above, I used a gut fermentation control diet plus various digestive aids, and I included milk thistle to assist Kevin's liver, which was clearly taking strain. I emphasised the importance of setting aside time to eat and to eat slowly and chew the food well. I also used grapefruit seed extract at the maximum dosage to treat the intestinal parasites, along with a multi-vitamin supplement, as many parasites can rob the body of important nutrients. *Giardia* in particular depletes your supplies of zinc and vitamin B complex, especially vitamin B_{12}.

Further history from Kevin revealed that he had taken antibiotics continuously over a two-year period for acne and he had also used numerous short courses for recurrent sore throats. This explained why the bacterial flora was so disturbed. He also told me that he had recurrent bouts of diarrhoea, which was explosive at times, a history that is very typical of intestinal parasites.

One month later Kevin was feeling a lot better in himself — more energy, less irritable, reduced sweating and feeling much lighter and brighter. The halitosis had improved, though it was not gone completely, and there was no hint of body odour anymore. His tongue was much improved but there was still some coating. His abdomen was still tender on examination and so I continued on Stage 1 of the gut fermentation control diet, as I was suspicious that the intestinal fermentation had not stopped.

Ultimately, there was a remarkable improvement in this young man, but it took all of four months to get the fermentation under control and to eliminate the parasites and kill the fungus. Despite being quite young he took time to improve, as shown by the stool tests we did at the end of each month. It was only after sixteen weeks that we got a completely normal stool result back. I have since asked him to be careful about his diet long-term and to take acidophilus capsules and garlic every day of his life.

Halitosis is a symptom of fermentation.

Kevin's case history is very interesting from a number of perspectives. Firstly, he did not present with intestinal symptoms. Rather, he had non-specific symptoms such as bad breath, body odour and heavy sweating. His bowel habit was in fact relatively normal except for the occasional bout of diarrhoea. In other words, a lack of abdominal symptoms does not mean that the intestines are normal. Many people are unaware of the fact that their gut is in trouble. This young man had multiple problems with the digestive tract — fermentation, parasites and a fungal infection.

Secondly, Kevin's medical history revealed the use of broad-spectrum antibiotics such as tetracycline, minocycline for his acne, as well as augmentin and orelox for the sore throats. As I have explained in my book *Alternatives to Antibiotics*, broad-spectrum antibiotics can wreak havoc in the intestine by disturbing the natural flora and allowing fungi to overgrow and allowing parasites to take hold.

Thirdly, the slow improvement indicated how chronic the problem really was; in other words, he had probably had intestinal disturbances for many years, long before the halitosis began to bother him.

Halitosis can also be associated with fever and with dental problems, but by far the commonest cause is gut fermentation.

So if you meet someone with halitosis, consider the possibility that there may be an intestinal disturbance.

CASE HISTORY — GARY: GURGLING SOUNDS

Gary was thirty-four and was married with three children. His wife complained that his tummy was always making gurgling sounds, which was most noticeable in bed at night. She also told him that he was extremely warm in bed, describing him as a radiator, radiating so much heat that it was uncomfortable to lie close to him. His wife had been telling him for a long time to go to a doctor for the overactive tummy sounds but he did not consider it serious enough. More recently, he began to get boils that were quite big and painful and some of them developed into abscesses, which had to be drained by the local GP.

Gary was convinced that there was nothing wrong with his digestive system, and when I suggested a possible link between his gurgling intestines and his skin condition he laughed and dismissed the idea as ludicrous. I told him I would bet that I was right and if the laboratory results came back as negative then I would refer him to another practitioner. He was willing to give it a try as he had nothing to lose.

When I examined him his rib-cage angle was approximately 120 degrees (30 degrees is normal) and he had obvious rib-cage humping. His abdomen was acutely tender on palpation and while listening to his abdomen it was clear that there was a significant intestinal disturbance, as I had never heard more active bowel sounds.

Gary lost the bet, as the urine revealed chemicals that indicated gross fermentation in the intestine. He still did not believe that this had anything to do with his boils and abscesses but was willing to give the treatment a trial of one month. His wife was very supportive and made sure that he ate only what was allowed on Stage 1 of the diet sheet. She also made sure that he took all the medication that I had given — digestive enzymes, magnesium oxide, mercurius solubilis in homeopathic form, caprylic acid and acidophilus capsules, plus garlic extract capsules.

One month later he was amazed at the results. The gurgling had stopped, his bowel habit had improved and he did not have one new boil in the month. He was so impressed that he now refers many people to me. I call him my agent, as he has referred so many people to me from the small town where he lives.

Active bowel sounds can be a symptom of fermentation.

What is interesting about this case history is the fact that Gary was producing so much heat from his body. When fermentation is well advanced, a lot of heat can be produced, which can be very uncomfortable. Gary told me that he preferred sleeping with only a sheet at night even though the temperature was low, and that he insisted on keeping the window open at night despite his wife complaining of the cold. Heat is a by-product of fermentation in much the same way that gas is.

So, if you hear of someone who is 'over-heating', think of fermentation as a possible cause.

CASE HISTORY — ANNA: RECURRENT CANDIDIASIS

Anna had been treated for both vaginal and intestinal thrush many times in the past but it kept recurring. When she came to me she was desperate for help to solve the problem, as the conventional drugs that she had been using were clearly not working. She had also been to a naturopath who treated her using the normal anti-candida diet along with probiotics and a range of anti-fungals, but the problem came back as soon as she stopped treatment. During the past fifteen years of practising natural medicine, I have had many patients like Anna who clearly did not respond to anti-candida treatment in the long term. When I encounter such a patient I am aware that there is another problem apart from intestinal candidiasis and that, whatever this problem is, it is disturbing the intestinal flora and not allowing it to correct permanently, resulting in the recurrence of the problem once treatment is stopped. Fermentation is the commonest underlying problem that I have found, and only when it is corrected first, followed by the correction of the flora, can a lasting cure be achieved.

Fermentation and putrefaction of food in the intestine leads to the production of nasty chemicals such as indican and putrescine, which inflame the intestinal wall. This inflammation must be corrected before the flora can normalise, as the nasty chemicals will continue to disturb the flora that reside in the crypts of the intestinal wall.

In Anna's case all I had to do was prove that I was dealing with yet another case of intestinal fermentation and treat it in the same way as the cases that I have mentioned earlier, that is with a special diet and digestive aids. This proved to be the case and when I had treated it and then corrected the intestinal bacterial flora Anna had a lasting improvement in her condition.

Recurrent candidiasis can be a symptom of fermentation.

So, if you are attending a doctor for the treatment of either vaginal or intestinal candidiasis and you are not getting anywhere, consider the possibility of fermentation.

CASE HISTORY — SINÉAD: EXHAUSTION UPON WAKING
Sinéad was eighteen years old when she came to me complaining of low energy. This is the commonest complaint I hear and it has many causes. Sinéad told me that she used to wake up most mornings feeling drugged and that it took her about an hour to 'come alive'. Her energy would dip in the afternoon and she often had to go to bed early in the evening as she felt tired. Because this kind of energy pattern is very unusual among teenagers, who tend to have a high natural energy, I proceeded to ask about other symptoms so that I could make a tentative diagnosis. After questioning her and examining her, I was unsure what the primary problem was. Investigations revealed that she had a low ferritin level, marginally low thyroid function, as well as intestinal fermentation. I treated the latter and gave her a

non-constipating iron supplement. Within one month her energy was back to normal. I advised her to continue with the treatment and, in the long term, not to eat her main meal late in the evening as she had been doing. She continued to improve over the following two months and was then able to maintain a good energy level throughout the day with no medication.

Low energy can be a symptom of fermentation.

This case history is very interesting for a number of reasons. Firstly, Sinéad's thyroid function returned to normal without being treated. I have found this with cases of intestinal dysbiosis as well. Hypothyroidism in many cases is secondary to some other condition in the body, and Sinéad exemplified this well.

Secondly, low energy may have more than one cause in the same patient, so it is important to look for multiple causes, including vitamin and mineral deficiencies (especially vitamin B_{12} and iron), low thyroid function, intestinal dysbiosis and intestinal fermentation.

Thirdly, the symptom of feeling hungover or drugged upon waking is a cardinal symptom of fermentation. If a person with a digestive disturbance is consuming sugar or sugary foods, the sugar may ferment and form alcohol. This alcohol is then absorbed across the intestinal wall and intoxicates the person — this is what is meant by the term 'auto-intoxication'. It means that toxic chemicals are being produced *inside* the body as distinct from chemicals that enter the body from outside.

Fermentation is a good example of how a normal body process (digestion) can go wrong and result in the production of toxins (alcohol, indican, putrescine). Auto-intoxication is the cause of a hungover or drugged feeling.

You have now learned the major symptoms associated with intestinal fermentation. Belching, increased bowel sounds and a hungover feeling are cardinal symptoms. You should suspect fermentation in anyone who is complaining of any of the symptoms displayed in Table 2.1.

Table 2.1 *SYMPTOMS OF FERMENTATION*

Abdominal	Non-Abdominal
Flatulence	Body odour
Bloating	Loss of interest
Nausea	Moodiness
Indigestion	Irritability
Halitosis	Headaches
Coated tongue	Cold peripheries
Gurgling sounds	Heavy sweating
	Urinary frequency

HOW FERMENTATION IS DIAGNOSED

A diagnosis of fermentation can be confirmed by means of a urine test. This urine test looks for the presence of a chemical called indican. If this chemical is present it strongly suggests that nasty chemicals, of which indican is one, are being produced in the body, absorbed into the bloodstream and excreted in the urine. However, basing a diagnosis on laboratory results alone is never correct; simply put, it is bad medicine.

In diagnosing a clinical condition such as fermentation in the digestive tract, I always take a history from the patient. The list of symptoms in Table 2.1 above can give an idea if fermentation is occurring or not. The next important step is to examine the patient from head to toe. I am shocked by the number of well-trained doctors who fail to do this. When I was at medical school, one of our professors, who was in his early eighties, used to say that the two best diagnostic tools a doctor has are his or her eyes and ears. Investigations are there merely to assist and nothing more.

Along with some of the symptoms mentioned in Table 2.1 above, I also look for some of the clinical signs on examination. This examination should include the facial skin, eyes, teeth and tongue, nails and palms of the hands, thyroid gland, blood pressure and pulse, abdomen and thorax, feet and ankles. I find it helpful to examine the neck, shoulders, mid-back and lower back as well if time permits and if the patient has symptoms relating to these areas.

Having listened to the patient's symptoms and having examined them top-to-toe, I now have an excellent impression of what is actually happening in this person's body to create their symptoms. I can then make a tentative or provisional diagnosis.

How Fermentation is Treated

Now that we know how fermentation is diagnosed, we come to the most important aspect of this condition and that is how to treat it.

There are two aspects to the treatment. Firstly, treating the condition itself, and secondly, helping the patient to understand and cope with the underlying cause, which in adults is often stress.

To treat the condition itself it is important to use both a diet and medicines that will support and heal the digestive tract. Firstly, let's deal with the diet.

GUT FERMENTATION CONTROL DIET

Table 2.2 illustrates the diet that I have used successfully for the past fifteen years.

Table 2.2 *GUT FERMENTATION CONTROL DIET*

This diet is in four stages, each lasting one month. Do not proceed to the next stage until you have been examined and re-tested. Do not stop any medicines that you have been prescribed in Stage 1 until you have seen your practitioner.

STAGE 1

This stage will last for one month approximately. Follow the diet strictly, as cheating may cause severe reactions, e.g. headache, diarrhoea. You may experience a detox reaction within the first week of commencing treatment; it is very important not to give up at this point. Eat only the following foods in Stage 1.

Meat	all sorts, including beef, venison, lamb. No processed meats.
Poultry	including chicken, turkey, guinea fowl. Try to use organic poultry.
Fish	not in batter.
Vegetables	all types except mushroom, sweetcorn and peas. Best steamed, stir fried or baked.
Fruit	pawpaw (papaya), rhubarb and grapefruit are the best to use
Salads	
Soups	do not add potato as it is too starchy
Cheese	excluding all soft cheese, e.g. cottage, cream cheeses
Live yoghurt	
Eggs	
Soya	soya milk, soya flour, tofu, miso, etc.

Herbal teas, e.g. lemon with some fresh lemon juice added
Olive oil and spices are okay

Drinks	only water and herbal teas

N.B. *Do not eat any starch — rice, pasta, potato, breads*
DO NOT GET CONSTIPATED!

STAGE 2

You should be feeling a lot better now. Try each of the following foods one at a time. Try each food for two to three days. If you tolerate it well, continue with it; if you cannot tolerate it yet, delete it from your diet for another month. Here is the list of foods to test:

Bread	must be yeast-free
Rice cakes	
Rye	Ryvita and yeast-free rye bread, e.g. sour-dough rye bread
Fruits	try each new fruit one at a time
Oats	
Dairy produce	
Rice	best forms are Basmati rice or brown rice

STAGE 3

In this stage you can add in yeast-containing foods.
Here is a list of yeast foods:

Breads	including rolls, croissants, pastry, doughnuts
Pickles	
Vinegar	
Alcohol	wine and beer are fermented and so contain yeast
Dried fruits	raisins, currants, sultanas, prunes, dates

Malted cereals and malted drinks (Horlicks, Ovaltine)
Mushrooms (they are a fungus)
Gravy mixes
Spreads
Yoghurts
Yeast, e.g. brewers yeast

STAGE 4

In this stage you can add in sugar-containing foods.
Jams/marmalades

Breakfast cereals	Cornflakes, Rice Crispies, etc.
Desserts/cakes/biscuits	
Soft drinks	Coca-Cola, Fanta, etc.

Sugar/confectionery/chocolate
Read labels and see that most processed foods contain sugars such as maltose, dextrose, sucrose, glucose, etc.

Let's look at each stage to give you an overview of the whole diet plan.

STAGE 1

As you will see from Stage 1 of this diet, there are many foods that have been excluded. These include all cereals, all forms of starch, most fruit — except for pawpaw (papaya) rhubarb and grapefruit, which are good for the digestive tract — all yeast products, and all sugar-containing products. The reason for removing sugar from the diet is because sugar will ferment to alcohol, adding to the toxic load on the body. Starch is removed to rest the digestive tract, as starchy, doughy foods are quite hard to digest and so increase the workload on a digestive tract that is already in difficulty. Fruits are excluded because they contain sugar.

So Stage 1 of the diet is aimed at minimising the workload on the digestive tract and excluding foods that will ferment easily, especially sugary foods. It also aims to exclude all yeast foods, as yeast is a necessary ingredient for fermentation to occur.

Constipation will delay improvement so it is important to use flaxseed oil or flaxseed oil capsules to ensure good elimination.

STAGE 2

After approximately one month on Stage 1, I reassess the patient. If the patient reports an improvement and if I find an improvement on examination, then I repeat the urine test to prove that the fermentation is indeed under control.

If the urine test confirms that there has been an improvement, I then ask the patient to experiment with the list of foods in Stage 2. The idea is to introduce each new food one at a time for a few days to see if it aggravates the condition or not. If there is no aggravation then it is safe to continue with it, but if there is doubt or if it clearly aggravates, then it must be excluded from the diet for another month at least. Because yeast-free bread is included in the list of foods in the second stage and because some people have a problem with gluten, which can be quite an irritant to the intestines, I ask my patients to put bread at the bottom of the list. From experience, bread (wheat or rye) is the food item most likely to cause an aggravation during the second stage.

So Stage 2 attempts to broaden the list of permitted foods to make the patient's life easier, while still excluding yeast foods (reintroduced in Stage 3) and sugary foods (Stage 4). Each food item in Stage 2 must be tried one at a time to assess its effect on the patient's digestive tract.

STAGE 3

This involves the reintroduction of yeast foods. It is very important to be one hundred per cent certain that the digestive tract is digesting food properly before going to Stage 3. This is achieved by killing off any yeast or fungal overgrowths in the intestine and by repeating the urine test once more. Yeast and fungal overgrowths can be diagnosed by doing a fungal culture on a stool sample. I generally ask for a microscopic examination of a stool sample as well as a fungal culture. I also ask to have the stool sample examined for parasites, as they are extraordinarily common in Africa; interestingly, they are not uncommon in Europe, so it is really worthwhile checking for them — Chapter 3 deals with this topic in more detail.

To kill off yeast or fungal overgrowths I use an array of medicines. The best substance that I have used to date is grapefruit seed extract — if the patient is an adult I use 12–15 drops three times daily in a glass of water. (I discuss anti-fungals in more detail in Chapter 7.) I tend to use these anti-yeast/anti-fungal medicines during the second stage of the diet if the overgrowth is mild to moderate; however, if it is a heavy overgrowth I introduce this medicine at the very beginning, i.e. at the beginning of Stage 1.

Only when I have repeated the urine and stool samples and am clinically satisfied that there has been an improvement will I allow the patient to begin eating yeast foods again. At this stage I ask patients to note down any foods that cause them an aggravation or a return of their original symptoms. If they have been able to maintain the improvement that they gained at the end of Stage 1 all the way through to the end of Stage 3, then it is safe to say that they have a much healthier digestive tract and that it is going to remain in good condition in the long term. Most people will have worked so hard to achieve such an improvement in their health that they are often reluctant to go to Stage 4 and reintroduce sugar and foods containing sugar. Since sugar is so detrimental to our health and since we get enough sugar from fruit and honey it is better to avoid sugar completely.

STAGE 4

This involves adding in sugar and foods containing sugar. Many processed foods have sugar hidden in them. For example, many breakfast cereals for sale in supermarkets will have sugar in them.

If you are able to introduce these foods as well to the diet then you will have completed the return to a completely normal diet where you are allowed to eat anything. It is, however, good common sense not to consume too much sugar on a daily basis since it is so damaging to one's health.

MEDICINES

Now that we have looked at the dietary aspect of the treatment for fermentation, let's take a look at the medicines that are used to assist the digestive function of the gastro-intestinal tract.

DIGESTIVE ENZYMES

Firstly, I tend to prescribe digestive enzymes to ensure that what is eaten during the first two months on this programme is actually digested effectively. I usually prescribe one or two capsules to be taken at the beginning of each meal, i.e. one capsule if it is a small meal and two capsules if it is a bigger meal. This medicine effectively takes the pressure off the pancreas, which is the organ that produces most of the digestive enzymes in the small intestine.

GENTIANA LUTEA (GENTIAN IS THE COMMON NAME)
This is a herbal remedy. I tend to use it in tincture form to ensure better absorption. It is a bitter herb and so is effective at stimulating the release of digestive enzymes. All bitter substances are used to assist the digestive function of the gastro-intestinal tract.

MAGNESIUM OXIDE
I tend to use magnesium salts such as magnesium oxide initially for the first few weeks to cleanse the whole digestive tract. This is a very important step, especially in people who have had a long-standing digestive problem. If using magnesium salts I recommend one level teaspoon in a large glass of lukewarm water with some lemon juice added. This is taken first thing in the morning on an empty stomach.

DEALING WITH THE UNDERLYING CAUSE
The third aspect of treating this condition involves dealing with the underlying cause, which is usually stress. I will discuss how stress affects the digestive tract later in Chapter 4. Also, Chapter 10 of my book *Alternatives to Antibiotics* covers the treatment of this condition effectively.

Now I am going to discuss a case history to illustrate the treatment of fermentation in more detail.

CASE HISTORY — SYLVIA: DETOXIFICATION REACTION
Sylvia came to see me having been diagnosed with spastic colon by her GP. A colonoscopy and gastroscopy had revealed nothing. She was complaining of abdominal bloating, flatulence and

excessive bowel sounds, as well as halitosis and a permanent thick white coating on her tongue. This latter symptom was the one that disturbed her the most and prompted her to come for help. My investigations revealed that there was intestinal fermentation as well as a heavy overgrowth of *Candida albicans*. I began by treating the fermentation as described above. During the first week of treatment she experienced a significant detoxification reaction. The detoxification symptoms included nausea, loss of appetite, severe lethargy, headache and sore legs. Her tongue had an even thicker coating and the halitosis got much worse. It was only in the second week of treatment that her symptoms began to improve. By the end of the first month the flatulence and bloating had disappeared, as had the halitosis and the coating on the tongue. However, her energy had improved very little. I explained that we had not treated the candidiasis and so her energy would not return to normal until we had.

I've included Sylvia's case to explain what a detoxification reaction is. When you withdraw from any drug, food or chemical that is damaging you (e.g. cigarettes, alcohol, caffeine) you can get withdrawal symptoms. In addition, when one has intestinal fermentation, nasty chemicals are being produced that are toxic to the body. It was only when Sylvia commenced the treatment that she realised just how toxic her body was. It is important to understand that when you treat the digestive tract you can feel much worse initially. This initial detox reaction can be so severe in some people that they have to give up — but it is worth remembering the saying: 'no pain, no gain'.

Having experienced detox reactions myself, I can understand why some people give up after a day or two. However, it helps to be aware that you may feel much worse and to prepare for it by taking time off work or doing it over a long weekend so that you can rest. Having the support of a sympathetic partner can make it that much easier.

LONG-TERM EFFECTS OF FERMENTATION ON YOUR WELL-BEING

Contamination of the body with toxic chemicals will eventually result in a build-up of metabolic wastes, as the detoxifying organs — liver and kidneys — become stressed and unable to function effectively. To get rid of these toxins the body dumps them into less important tissues such as the skin, connective tissue, muscles and joints, in an attempt to protect the vital organs — heart, liver, kidneys, etc. In the less important tissues, if these deposits of toxins continue, the cells will begin to function with difficulty, and disease will become manifest. In the skin, this can produce skin rashes, broken blood vessels and age spots; in the connective tissue it can result in wrinkling of the skin and flaccidity; in the muscles it can result in rheumatism, and in the joints arthrosis and arthritis.

If this contamination of the body continues untreated for years, the vital organs will also become affected, thereby compromising one's health much more obviously. This process manifests itself in the blood vessels as arteriosclerosis, in the gall-bladder as gall-stones, in the kidney as urinary frequency, renal stones and gravel, in the heart as angina and ultimately infarction, and in the liver as fatty degeneration.

If the brain is compromised, poorly nourished brain cells will lead to poor short-term memory, poor concentration, irritability and depression. The thought processes become slower, and ultimately melancholia and depression become apparent. The mental and emotional well-being of the entire person is eventually affected. They are then then caught in a cycle of negativity which is reversible only through a prolonged detoxification, coupled with medicinal support for the main organs that are in difficulty.

Now you can understand why so many health practitioners around the world insist on detoxification and why so many health spas around the world are full of people who will testify to the benefits of treatment. Many patients will do a three-day detoxification once a month and then a major detoxification for three weeks once a year. For most people this is sufficient, but some require longer periods of treatment. Women tend to avail of these treatments more than men do — in general women take their health more seriously — but anyone who detoxifies regularly will stay younger for longer, their skin will be clearer and their weight more stable.

So, if you wish to delay the ageing process and prevent degenerative diseases such as rheumatism and arthritis, detoxify on a monthly basis and check for fermentation in the digestive tract and treat it if present.

SUMMARY

Fermentation is a common disorder of the digestive system. It means that food is not being digested efficiently. The commonest cause in an adult is unquestionably stress. Stress upsets the digestive tract, making it difficult to digest and absorb the food effectively.

Abdominal symptoms of this condition include flatulence, bloating, halitosis, nausea, indigestion and increased bowel sounds. Fermentation affects your whole body and your whole being; the non-abdominal symptoms include heavy sweating, cold hands and feet, body odour, urinary frequency and headache. Your mental well-being can also be affected significantly and can cause symptoms such as apathy, moodiness and irritability.

Fermentation is diagnosed by means of a urine test and is treated with a strict diet, which excludes all foods containing starch, sugar and yeast, and with medication to assist the digestive process. The initial few days of treatment can involve a detoxification reaction during which you may feel worse; however, it does not last longer than one week.

It is critically important to diagnose and to treat intestinal fermentation as it can have long-term consequences on your physical, mental and emotional well-being. If you have the symptoms or signs of fermentation as I have described them above, go to a practitioner of natural medicine and have your urine tested; most family doctors do not know how to diagnose or to treat this condition. If you have the condition, follow the treatment guidelines that I have recommended.

3

DYSBIOSIS

The skin, the digestive tract (from mouth to anus), and the vagina in females, are colonised by billions of bacteria which are essential for the proper functioning of these organs. In medical terms these billions of bacteria are referred to as the body's bacterial flora. They live both on our skin and inside us. The greatest number of bacteria are found in the digestive tract, where up to five hundred different species reside. Collectively, these bacteria are referred to as the intestinal flora. The intestinal flora are responsible for numerous important activities, some of which are closely linked to immune function, nutritional status and detoxification of the body.

The quality of our intestinal flora is determined by the balance between the various species of bacteria. Each species keeps the others in check, preventing the overgrowth of any one species. The ecological balance can be disturbed by certain factors such as diet, chronic stress, surgery, major temperature changes and drugs (such as antibiotics). If, for example, the body's bacterial flora are partly destroyed by taking an antibiotic, harmful bacteria can replace the 'good' bacteria that have been destroyed. Certain antibiotics, like amoxycillan, can upset the bacterial flora of the bowel and vagina. In both of these regions, a yeast infection called thrush, which is caused by *Candida albicans*, can develop. A thrush infection is more apparent in the vagina as a visible discharge; it is less apparent in the bowel, as little or no symptoms are initially present.

In a healthy person, 'good' bacteria, such as those found in live yoghurt (acidophilus and bifidus), produce acids, such as lactic acid, which keep the environment around them acidic. Harmful bacteria and yeast, such as those responsible for thrush, cannot grow when the environment becomes more acidic. This can happen when certain drugs are taken (antibiotics and the contraceptive pill in particular). These drugs alter the natural bacterial flora lining the digestive and genital tracts, which can result in a chronic infection of these organs with harmful bacteria, yeast or fungi.

'Good' bacteria play a very important role in digestion. For example, the higher the percentage of these 'good' bacteria in the digestive tract, the more peristalsis (natural contractions of the bowel) is stimulated. Peristalsis flushes out waste material in the stool.

The nature of the bacterial population in the intestine has been shown to have a greater effect on bowel habit than the addition of dietary fibre. The medical profession has latched onto bran as the most important dietary factor in the management of many bowel problems. However, while I was still a medical student, the link between cancer of the colon and disturbances in the bacterial population of the bowel had already been clearly established.

DYSBIOSIS

When the ecological balance of healthy bacteria in the digestive tract is disturbed, we call this dysbiosis. It implies that some of the good bacteria have been killed off by drugs such as antibiotics or by stress or by poor diet, and that bad bacteria have taken their place.

Dr Metchnikoff was the person who first used this term back at the beginning of the twentieth century. Dr Metchnikoff, who succeeded Louis Pasteur as director of the famous Pasteur Institute in Paris, suggested that many digestive diseases resulted from dysbiosis. He maintained that digestive disturbances such as peptic ulcers, diarrhoea, constipation and even cancer of the colon were all the end result of disturbances in the ecology of the bacterial population in the digestive tract. He won a Nobel Prize for his work on the bacterial flora of the digestive tract in 1908.

Dysbiosis means there is an abnormal bacterial population in the digestive tract; it means that there is an overgrowth of a bacterium such as staphylococcus or an overgrowth of a yeast or fungus such as *Candida albicans.*

So dysbiosis is really an ecological imbalance in the digestive tract.

The symptoms associated with dysbiosis are varied and depend on which type of dysbiosis one has and which bacteria/fungus has overgrown. According to the book *Digestive Wellness* by Elizabeth Lepski, there are four different kinds of dysbiosis.

PUTREFACTION DYSBIOSIS

This is where the protein part of our diet is not digested properly and so it putrefies, producing very toxic chemicals and gases. This leads to bloating, indigestion and fatigue. In people with putrefaction dybiosis, some bad bacteria, *Bacteriodes spp.*, overgrow. The bacteriodes break down the vitamin B_{12} consumed in food, thereby rendering the body deficient in B_{12}. This results in symptoms such as fatigue, depression, tingling in the hands and feet. These bacteria also convert bile into nasty chemicals associated with bowel cancer.

Putrefaction dysbiosis is particularly common in people who eat lots of protein, such as meat, eggs, gluten in flour and breads, and milk products.

FERMENTATION DYSBIOSIS

This is when there is an overgrowth of yeast such as *Candida albicans* — yeast is a fungus. For any fermentation process, as people who manufacture wine and beer will know, one needs a carbohydrate such as fruit, sugar or starch (breads, potato, and pasta). So people with this type of dysbiosis tend to eat too much carbohydrate and tend to have a yeast overgrowth in the digestive tract. They also suffer from bloating, fatigue, depression and all the other symptoms mentioned in the last chapter.

DEFICIENCY DYSBIOSIS
This is where a course of antibiotics, for example, has rendered the body deficient in beneficial good bacteria. Because the good bacteria are our first line of defence, those affected are prone to infections, allergies, parasites and IBS.

SENSITISATION DYSBIOSIS
This is when the digestive tract becomes highly sensitive to certain foods and chemicals. People with this type of dysbiosis find that their energy drops after eating certain foods and tend to have symptoms not associated with the digestive tract, e.g. inflamed joints, skin rashes, etc. They can go on to develop auto-immune diseases such as rheumatoid arthritis, eczema and SLE (systemic lupus erythematosis).

SYMPTOMS ASSOCIATED WITH DYSBIOSIS
The symptoms of dysbiosis are best described by means of case histories.

CASE HISTORY — JACK: ITCHY SKIN RASH
Jack was twenty-five years old and came to see me because of a rash on his scrotum and in his armpits. It had appeared quite suddenly and was spreading. He found it intensely itchy and although scratching relieved it, he often had rebound itchiness more intense than before. He found that the rash waxed and waned, in that it would be quite intense for a few days and then would heal, only to become worse again. He had tried various creams from his local GP, all to no avail.

When I questioned him further, he said that he also suffered from diarrhoea and constipation and that his stool did not seem quite normal, in that it was poorly formed. He also complained of passing water quite frequently, especially in the morning. His energy was low and his siblings described him as moody.

On examining him, the skin rash was quite inflamed and angry-looking and was spread across both armpits; it had a raised edge to it. The scrotal rash spread along the inner leg and buttocks towards the anus. He then told me that he suffered from anal itching on occasion.

Stool and urine tests revealed an overgrowth of two species of fungi, *Geotrichium spp.* and *Candida spp.* I suspected that the skin rash was fungal in origin and therefore treated him using anti-fungal drops, i.e. grapefruit seed extract, as well as a probiotic and a multi-vitamin supplement along with a diet excluding all sugar and yeast. I also recommended using an anti-fungal cream on the rash itself, e.g. tea tree oil.

Within six weeks of following this course of treatment the rash was gone, his energy had improved and he felt much healthier. A repeat stool test showed the presence of only one fungus, *Geotrichium spp.*, and so I continued treatment for a further six weeks until the stool sample was clear.

Skin rashes are not uncommon when a fungal overgrowth in the digestive tract becomes systemic, i.e. spreads to other parts of the body. Some of the strangest skin rashes that I have seen over the years have been associated with fungal infections. I know this because when I treat the intestinal dysbiosis the rash disappears.

Fungal skin infections have a predilection for moist areas of the body — groin, armpits, between the toes — but are by no means limited to these areas. Classic ringworm can occur anywhere.

If you suffer from skin itching or if you have an unusual rash, consider having a stool analysis done.

Skin rashes can be a symptom of intestinal dysbiosis.

CASE HISTORY — JAMES: PUFFY EYES

James was forty-two years old and woke up every morning with bags under his eyes. His face looked old and puffy and he never woke up refreshed but always tired. He was worried about getting old, although he was still in his early forties and was otherwise quite healthy. He found that the puffiness usually cleared within an hour or two, but if he ate bread or pastry or anything with flour his eyes would get puffy shortly afterwards. His energy was good during the morning, dipped a bit in the afternoon, especially if he had a big lunch, and picked up in the evening. He said that of late he noticed a very strong odour when he passed a bowel motion and when he passed wind. These symptoms had been there for approximately six months.

His stool result showed a 3+ overgrowth of yeast and a 2+ overgrowth of *Candida albicans* on fungal culture. He clearly had intestinal dysbiosis and was beginning to get fermentation dysbiosis — he ate his main meal in the evening and it then fermented in his digestive tract overnight. This is why he felt so groggy in the mornings and why his face and eyes were puffy.

I decided to use a gut fermentation control diet in this case, as well as probiotics, a good multi-vitamin supplement and antifungal and digestive enzymes. Within a month of treatment he had improved but had difficulty sticking to the diet as he loved starchy food — bread, rice, pasta, potato.

CASE HISTORY — SARAH: ERRATIC VISION

Sarah had enjoyed excellent health all her life but in the past few months she noticed that her visual acuity was deteriorating. She was thirty-nine and had always had excellent vision so she never wore glasses. About six months prior to her visit she noticed that she was unable to read printed material that she previously had no problem with. She used the term 'blurred vision', as she found that she could not focus as well as before. She found that her vision was not blurred continuously but only intermittently. She therefore decided to go to her GP, who then referred her to an eye specialist. After a battery of tests he could find nothing wrong with her. As the problem was getting worse, a few months later she decided to seek help again and ended up on my doorstep.

I did my investigations and they were all normal except the stool analysis, which revealed mild intestinal dysbiosis. I treated her accordingly and within one month she noticed that her visual acuity had improved remarkably. She was grateful that there was nothing seriously wrong with her eyes and was now aware of how to treat it if it ever recurred again in the future.

Sarah's case is very interesting in that she did not present with digestive symptoms or with fatigue, but rather a visual problem. Her vision was very important to her as she was a legal secretary and had to read and type documents as part of her work. She was proud of her ability to read small text and so was shocked to find that her vision was beginning to fail her. Many people had dismissed this as an age-related deterioration in her eyesight, but because her mother was seventy-five and still had excellent vision Sarah was adamant that there was a cause for it. How right she proved to be!

Old age and ill health do not go hand-in-hand. The man who taught me a lot of natural medicine in Austria was seventy-seven years old and he was embarrassingly healthy. He taught me that the ageing process is intimately related to intestinal toxicity. 'The digestive tract is the most toxic part of the body', he used to say. After fifteen years of practice I can only agree with him. If you keep it in good condition it will supply you with good nutrition; to assist it do regular fasts to help it get rid of toxic build-ups. Look after the digestive tract and you will have excellent health.

Erratic vision can be a symptom of dysbiosis.

CASE HISTORY — SEÁN: IRRITABILITY

Seán's wife asked him to come and see me as he became quite irritable if he went for long periods of time without eating; he also became irritable after eating sugary foods, especially chocolate.

He was becoming hard to live with and his wife was worried that he might have diabetes.

Blood and urine tests revealed that he was not diabetic but rather that he was suffering from bouts of hypoglycaemia or low blood sugar level. If the blood sugar level drops too low it can disturb the central nervous system, causing irritability; it is usually associated with dysbiosis. I did a stool analysis, and sure enough he had a 3+ overgrowth of a fungus species, *Mucor spp.* In Seán's case it was necessary to use a pancreatic remedy as well the normal treatment for dysbiosis, which I shall discuss later in this chapter.

After three months of treatment he was no longer suffering from bouts of hypoglycaemia but his stool sample still had a 1+ overgrowth of *Mucor spp.* I then decided to send him for colonic irrigation to clean out the colon and to instil a probiotic into the colon. After three sessions the stool result was back to normal. He found the colonic irrigation so helpful that he now has a maintenance treatment once a month.

Why do people with dysbiosis suffer from hypoglycaemia? The answer requires a bit of explanation. Fungal overgrowths in the intestinal tract demand sugar in any form — table sugar, sweets, chocolate.

As a result, people with intestinal dysbiosis tend to eat lots of foods containing sugar. Eating foods rich in refined sugar causes high levels of glucose to enter the bloodstream rapidly. This puts stress on the pancreas, which is then forced to release large quantities of insulin to lower the blood sugar level. These ups and downs in the blood sugar level when sugary foods are eaten not only stress the pancreas but also disturb the adrenal glands. Sometimes in these ups and downs the blood sugar level drops too low; this is how hypoglycaemia occurs. The solution is to avoid sugars completely.

Hypoglycaemia is not uncommon. It produces symptoms such as irritability, cold sweats, shaky hands, a hollow feeling in the stomach and a need to eat something quickly. If you suffer from these symptoms, avoid all foods containing refined carbohydrates and consult your practitioner.

Irritability can be a symptom of dysbiosis.

CASE HISTORY — KAREN: CONSTANT TIREDNESS

Karen was thirty-three years old and in the prime of her life. She had a successful career, was happily married with one child and was very pleased with her life. She loved exercise but found that she did not have the energy anymore. She woke up tired, yawned all day, could fall asleep in the afternoon if she had the chance, and arrived home in the evening exhausted. Her general health was fine but of late she found that she was getting severe pre-menstrual symptoms — moodiness, bloating, headaches and breast tenderness — which she had not experienced before. She also found that her period was less regular, in that her cycle had lengthened from 28 days to 32 days. She had also gained four kilograms in weight over a three-month period.

On examining Karen, I noticed that she had a distinctive body odour and some of her toenails had a fungal infection; she also had a touch of athlete's foot. Her abdomen was distended and tender in places when pressed on. The hormonal blood tests, including her thyroid function, were all normal, as were the stool and urine tests. What to do next?

Well, my clinical suspicion was that she had dysbiosis with possible hypothyroidism (low thyroid function), as this would explain all of her symptoms, yet the investigations did not confirm it.

When I am confronted with this situation I always go with my gut feeling (no pun intended). I therefore treated her as if she had dysbiosis and decided to observe her symptoms. She showed an instant improvement and her energy increased steadily throughout the period of treatment. In addition I used a thyroid gland extract, as I was suspicious that she had sub-clinical hypothyroidism. I also prescribed a high-potency vitamin B complex and magnesium supplement.

Karen's case is interesting in that medical tests do not always confirm a clinical diagnosis. According to the laboratory tests she did not have hypothyroidism or dysbiosis. Yet in retrospect it is obvious that she did have both of these conditions. Basing a medical diagnosis on medical investigations is wrong, as you can see from Karen's case. A diagnosis should be based on the history and examination.

Sub-clinical hypothyroidism is when the thyroid gland becomes underactive, resulting in a feeling of tiredness and depression, along with weight gain; however, the hormonal levels are not low enough to be abnormal on blood tests. This condition is probably one of the most under-diagnosed medical problems. In other words, even if the blood tests are normal, it does not necessarily mean that the gland is functioning properly.

For a woman, a vitamin B complex supplement is very important, especially if she is on the contraceptive pill, is pregnant or has been under stress. The B vitamins and magnesium are essential to release energy from food.

$$\text{FOOD} \xrightarrow{\text{B complex}}_{\text{magnesium}} \text{ENERGY}$$

Vitamin B complex and magnesium are also essential for the production of serotonin, a neurotransmitter in the brain and the digestive tract. Insufficient B vitamins and magnesium can lead to depression, becuase not enough serotonin can be produced — serotonin is described as the 'feel good' chemical.

How do you become deficient in vitamin B complex when you develop dysbiosis?

The good bacteria that line the digestive tract manufacture a number of B vitamins which our bodies can utilise. When these good bacteria are killed off, with antibiotics for example, we can easily become deficient in one or more of the B vitamins. In addition, bad microbes such as yeast or fungi or *Bacteriodes spp*. can use some of the B vitamins that we consume in our food; parasites in the bowel can also do this. Hence, anyone with dysbiosis can become deficient in certain vitamins and minerals. So, if you have dysbiosis take a good vitamin/mineral supplement.

CASE HISTORY — BRIAN: FEELING SPACEY

Brian was twenty-eight years old and was worried that there was something wrong with him. During the last year he had been having difficulty concentrating and his short-term memory was letting him down to the point where he had to write everything down. Most disturbing for him was what he described as feeling 'a bit spacey', where his thinking was not clear. He was young and had never experienced such symptoms before and was convinced that he had a brain tumour or some other malevolent disease. Extensive tests by his GP and a consultant neurologist revealed nothing, and they suggested that he see a psychiatrist. He was unhappy with this suggestion, but because he was desperate, he agreed and went along to the psychiatrist. The latter could find nothing wrong with him either and suggested that he was malingering and referred him back to his GP. It was at this point that he came to see me.

Since feeling spacey is a cardinal symptom of dysbiosis, which many conventional doctors fail to diagnose, and since Brian had other symptoms and signs suggestive of dysbiosis, I had a stool analysis done, which did indeed reveal fermentation dysbiosis as well as abnormal liver function.

I treated the dysbiosis and gave him milk thistle to assist his liver. Not only did all his symptoms disappear but his memory and concentration returned to normal and he no longer needed to write himself notes.

How does dysbiosis cause these symptoms? Fermentation results in toxic chemicals being produced that not only impair liver function but also interfere with brain function; hence the symptoms of memory loss and lack of concentration as well as the strange symptom of feeling spacey, which is really a symptom of auto-intoxication (where toxins are produced inside the body instead of being consumed in food or drink).

CASE HISTORY — MARIANNE: PHLEGMY COUGH

Marianne was fourteen years old and had a constant cough with lots of phlegm. Sometimes the phlegm was so thick that she felt her airway was going to block. She was very worried about getting colds or 'flu, because these worsened her condition and she was then afraid to sleep at night because she felt she was going to suffocate. She also said that she had lots of wax in her ears and had to use wax softener on occasions to clear them. There was mucus in her stool on a few occasions as well. All in all a very mucusy child! She also told me that she was addicted to milk, chocolate and sweets.

On examining her I noticed that she had an acidic rash on her face and arms and had the early signs of acne on her forehead. She had a white coating on her tongue, her abdomen was a little tender in places and when I listened to her chest it sounded normal. The tests revealed dysbiosis. I suspected then that she was reacting to certain foods in her diet, especially the mucus-forming foods — sugar, dairy foods, chocolate.

Because she did not have regular bowel motions, I sent her for colonic irrigation while treating the dysbiosis. After two months of treatment her skin looked much better and she told me that her energy was excellent and that she now had a regular well-formed bowel motion; however, the cough was not gone, despite having improved. I then decided to exclude all dairy produce from the diet as well, and one month later the cough was gone.

Marianne's case illustrates the connection between the digestive and respiratory tracts. There are two main supply-tubes in the body — the respiratory tract, which supplies air, and the digestive tract, which supplies food. Because both of these tubes are exposed to the outside world — in fact they are really an interface between the outside environment and the internal environment of the body — they have to be protected, as they are located inside the human body. Both tubes are lined with billions of bacteria called the bacterial flora. These bacteria protect the body from harmful bacteria and so they constitute the first line of defence of the immune system. Disturbances in the bacterial flora can therefore have significant effects on one's health. These effects are not just limited to the digestive tract; they can be seen in the respiratory tract, the skin and the vagina. In Marianne's case, the respiratory tract was the main source of difficulty, but it is obvious from her history that the skin and digestive tract were also involved, though to a lesser extent.

If the digestive or respiratory tract become infected or exposed to harmful or irritating chemicals, they produce mucus as a form of protection. For example, if you get a cold, your nose produces lots of mucus. If both tracts are producing mucus then it is most likely that the patient has dysbiosis.

Marianne had suffered from recurrent ear infections when she was younger and had been given many courses of antibiotics. These drugs had probably damaged the bacterial flora in her body.

Marianne's case is also interesting in that it illustrates the point that many people with dysbiosis have food intolerances. It was clear that Marianne had a dairy intolerance, as indicated by the improvement when it was excluded from her diet. It is important to always check for food intolerances, especially to wheat and dairy products, but in some patients one must check for all the gluten cereals — wheat, rye, oats and barley.

All in all, Marianne's case was both interesting and informative.

A chronic cough can be a symptom of dysbiosis.

Case History — Paula: Headaches

Paula was twenty-two years old and was suffering from severe headaches. She said that the headaches felt like a pressure sensation inside her head and in the back of her eyes. On occasion the headaches were accompanied by a feeling of weakness and nausea. She had them approximately two or three times a week, and although painkillers did help she was worried about having to take them so frequently. The headaches were also interfering with her quality of life. Her GP had carried out numerous tests but they were all negative. Since she had been suffering like this for over a year, she decided to come to me for help.

When I examined her there was a lot of tension in her neck muscles and in her upper back. I was not sure whether this was the cause of her headaches and so I referred her for remedial massage while I was waiting for the results of her tests. The stool test revealed a 2+ overgrowth of *Candida albicans* in fungal form. I explained to her that dysbiosis can cause toxic headaches and that the description of her headaches sounded more like toxicity than tension headaches. I suggested that she treat the dysbiosis for a period of six weeks initially to see if it helped. It was three months later when I saw her again. I got a big hug from her as she was ecstatic that her headaches had gone two weeks after beginning treatment and had not returned.

Paula's case illustrates how toxic one can become when one has dysbiosis. I am sure that you have seen mould growing on food that has been exposed for too long. Moulds or fungi have roots that extend down into the bread. Well, when fungi grow on the intestinal wall they develop roots, called mycelia, that extend across the wall into the bloodstream. All the fungal waste products are then dumped into the bloodstream. Dysbiosis can also end up causing fermentation or putrefaction, releasing very toxic chemicals into the bloodstream, which can cause severe headaches.

So, if you suffer from recurrent headaches, find the underlying cause rather than taking painkillers — these only add to the toxic load. Get checked out to see if you have dysbiosis.

Headaches can be a symptom of dysbiosis.

OTHER SYMPTOMS OF DYSBIOSIS

So far, you have learned some of the minor symptoms of dys-biosis, such as skin rash, puffy eyes, erratic vision and so on. The cardinal symptoms of dysbiosis, however, are abdominal in nature. The following case history will illustrate some of these.

CASE HISTORY — DAVID: DIARRHOEA

David ran a grocery store and had to work long hours. He was thirty-three years old and was married with two children. He had been suffering from diarrhoea on and off for a few years. The stool was poorly formed most of the time and on occasion became very loose and had mucus in it. As he had a lot of perianal itching as well, he was convinced that he had worms. After two doses of worm medicine from his doctor he found that he still had the symptoms and so sought help from me. On questioning David he told me that he had been on tetracycline, an antibiotic, for about three years in his early twenties to treat acne; when he was much younger he had been on steroids and an occasional antibiotic for asthma.

In addition to having diarrhoea, he also complained of abdominal bloating and lots of wind, which embarrassed him.

A stool test revealed two species of fungus as well as mucus. In David's case I began treatment with colonic irrigation because of the high level of mucus in the stool sample. A probiotic was instilled into the colon after each treatment. I then treated the dysbiosis and gave him linseed oil (also called flaxseed oil) cap-sules to help bulk the stool and assist bowel clearance.

After two months of treatment David had a normal, well-formed stool and no bloating or wind for the first time in years. His digestive tract was well on the way to recovery.

This case illustrates well the abdominal symptoms associated with dysbiosis. A loose stool is common with this condition, although some people have constipation and others alternate between constipation and diarrhoea. Most people do not seek help when the consistency of the stool varies like this; they often dismiss it as due to dietary changes, etc. It is only if the symptoms become severe that they seek help. Bloating and flatulence are also common symptoms of dysbiosis, but again are usually not severe enough to warrant medical attention.

Other abdominal symptoms include abdominal cramps and, less commonly, abdominal pain. Indigestion is another symptom and is usually associated with a food intolerance, especially to wheat.

In summary then, intestinal dysbiosis can give rise to abdominal and non-abdominal symptoms, which I have listed below in Table 3.1.

Table 3.1 *SYMPTOMS OF DYSBIOSIS*

Abdominal Symptoms	Non-Abdominal Symptoms
Flatulence	Tiredness, Skin rash
Bloating	Irritability, Headache
Cramps or pain	Moodiness, Feeling spacey
Diarrhoea	Erratic vision, Vaginal discharge
Constipation	Menstrual problems, Prostatitis
Nausea	Puffy eyes, Pruritis*
	Poor memory
	Lack of concentration
	Urinary frequency

*pruritis means skin itching

Table 3.2 below shows the cardinal or major symptoms associated with dysbiosis.

Table 3.2 *CARDINAL SYMPTOMS OF DYSBIOSIS*

Lack of energy
Moodiness
Irritability
Change in bowel habit
Abdominal bloating

How Dysbiosis is Diagnosed

The simplest method of diagnosing this condition is on the basis of the patient's history and clinical examination. This is usually sufficient for any experienced practitioner.

To confirm one's clinical suspicions it may be necessary to order tests. The stool analysis test is the one that I have found to be the most reliable over the past fifteen years. However, a negative stool test does not mean that the patient's bacterial flora is normal. The piece of stool that was used for the test may not have had any abnormal levels of bacteria or yeast or may not have had fungi present, or it may have been left for too long or the laboratory may have made an error; there are many reasons why the result may not be representative of the patient's bacterial flora. When doing a stool analysis I also ask to have it checked for parasites, blood and mucus.

There are many other diagnostic tests, including blood tests, but these are usually not necessary provided that the practitioner is experienced and has a good laboratory to do the stool analysis.

How Dysbiosis is Treated

There is a lot of controversy about how to treat this condition. Books may vary somewhat as to specific treatment, but the principles of treatment are basically the same. The four main principles of treatment are as follows:

1. Do not feed the bad bacteria — diet is very important.
2. Kill off the bad bacteria — there are a range of antimicrobials on the market.

3. Replace the good bacteria — probiotics such as acidophilus.
4. Restore lost nutrients — a vitamin/mineral supplement.

Let's now examine each of these aspects of treatment in detail.

1. DIET

Some books suggest eliminating sugary foods only, while other books suggest eliminating foods containing yeast as well. Some practitioners also restrict wheat and dairy produce because some patients cannot tolerate these foods. Still other practitioners restrict all foods containing gluten (wheat, rye, oats and barley). What to do as regards diet then if you have dysbiosis? The answer lies with your own body. By testing different foods you will find out which foods are having a negative effect on your health.

I would advise following Stage 1 of the gut fermentation diet for one month and then adding in foods in Stage 2 only after you have tested them one at a time; if any of these foods cause a negative reaction, such as a drop in energy or abdominal bloating or indigestion, omit this food from your diet. It is important to try each of these new foods in Stage 2, one at a time and for two days at least. The yeast-free bread and the dairy produce are the foods most likely to cause a reaction. Do not go to Stage 3 until you have completed at least three months of treatment, or until the stool analysis is normal and there are no more symptoms of dysbiosis.

In summary, your diet should consist of all the foods in Stage 1, plus any foods in Stage 2 that you tolerate well. You are allowed rice as the main form of starch — brown rice and basmati rice are the best forms to use.

To put this another way, you must avoid sugar and all foods with sugar, avoid yeast-containing foods, moulds and fermented products, avoid cereals as well as dried fruit. The best source of help about what is and is not allowed is a good cookbook such as the *Beat Candida Cookbook* by Erica White.

2. ANTI-FUNGAL TREATMENT

Killing off the bad bacteria is a critical aspect of treatment. Some people believe that it is sufficient to treat dysbiosis with diet alone; others believe that diet plus taking a pro-biotic such as acidophilus is necessary to treat dysbiosis. However, the single most important aspect of treatment is to rid the body of the 'bad' microbes.

There are two main anti-microbials used by practitioners of natural medicine. The more potent of the two is grapefruit seed extract. Its advantage is that it is not just anti-fungal, it is also anti-parasitic and anti-viral. It can therefore be used almost regardless of the type of dysbiosis and regardless of the type of parasite. Its main disadvantage is its very bitter taste. Even when it is well diluted it is still very bitter and this makes it hard for some people to take. A way around this is to use it in capsule form. The dosage of liquid grape-fruit seed extract to use is fifteen drops two or three times daily, but even if you take it in capsule form make sure to take a glass of water with it.

The second anti-microbial that is used to treat dysbiosis is a substance called caprylic acid, a fatty acid that occurs naturally in coconuts. It has proven anti-fungal activity and the calcium and the magnesium salt — calcium caprylate and magnesium caprylate — survive the digestive juices of the stomach and small intestine and so can act on the large intestine or colon. Since most forms of dysbiosis involve the overgrowth of yeast or the growth of fungi within the colon, caprylic acid is a very useful medicine for this condition. The dosage varies with the strength of capsule. Use 400 mg capsules and start with one capsule daily for the first week, then one capsule twice daily for the second week and continue increasing the daily dosage at weekly intervals until you get to six capsules daily, which is the maximum dosage. Continue at this dosage until the stool analysis is normal. However, having said that, it is really best done with the help of your practitioner. Killing off fungi in the digestive tract can increase toxicity in the body if they are not eliminated promptly, and this is really where colonic irrigation can be so helpful, as it guarantees the elimination of dead fungi.

3. PROBIOTICS

The ecological balance of the intestinal flora can be restored back to normal by taking lots of good bacteria, either as live yoghurt or as a probiotic supplement. Probiotics are supplements that contain a number of species of good bacteria, e.g. *Lactobacillus acidophilus* and *Bifidobacterium bifidus* — some people refer to these two species as 'A' for acidophilus and 'B' for bifidus. Probiotic supplements are prepared as freeze-dried capsules or as powder. When water is added to the capsule or powder, the bacteria are regenerated and can multiply. It is important to store a probiotic supplement in the fridge after it has been opened. The dosage will depend on the degree of disturbance to your flora and so is best determined by your practitioner. A good maintenance dosage would be one or two capsules twice daily or the equivalent in powder form.

Healthfood shops have lots of probiotic supplements to choose from. Some of these are dairy-free for people sensitive to dairy produce. The more modern probiotic supplements may also contain what is called a prebiotic. There are two main prebiotics, inulin and fructo-oligosaccharide, which is abbreviated to FOS. These two compounds are food for the good bacteria and ensure their survival in the digestive tract. FOS or inulin can be taken alone or in combination with a probiotic supplement. FOS and inulin are excellent substances but they can cause a lot of flatulence, so slowly increase the dosage.

Live yoghurt or a probiotic should be used daily by everyone, because every day we are constantly losing good bacteria from the digestive tract, in the same way that we shed skin every day. Probiotics are essential in the treatment of dysbiosis.

4. *RESTORE LOST NUTRIENTS*

Good bacteria are important for many reasons, one of which is that they manufacture some of the B vitamins that help your body to function effectively. Loss of these good bacteria results in a loss of these essential vitamins. Often bad bacteria and parasites then colonise the digestive tract and rob you of essential vitamins and minerals. Hence, a good high-potency vitamin and mineral supplement is essential when helping the body to recover from dysbiosis. There are many good vitamin/mineral supplements on the market today. Your health practitioner will advise what is available in your local area.

SUMMARY

Intestinal dysbiosis is a condition of epidemic proportions in the West and in urban areas of the developing world. It has huge effects on one's overall health as it can affect many parts of the body, not just the digestive tract. If you have suffered from chronic stress, been traumatised, been on antibiotics or the contraceptive pill, you might well have this condition. It can be diagnosed clinically on the basis of a person's symptoms — some practitioners use a question-naire — and what signs one has on examination by a health practitioner. This diagnosis can then be confirmed by doing a stool analysis. Treatment of this condition involves the use of a diet, probiotics, anti-fungal medication and a vitamin/mineral supplement.

4

HOW STRESS AFFECTS THE DIGESTIVE SYSTEM

The life of a modern city-dweller can be quite stressful. John is twenty-five years old and lives in Dublin. John wakes up at eight o'clock on weekdays and gets ready for work. As the traffic can be very heavy, he tends to skip breakfast and heads straight for the office. On arriving at work he has a cup of strong coffee to kickstart his body into action. Mid-morning he usually has a muffin or a biscuit with another cup of coffee. He works in the sales division of a large computer company and is always under great pressure, with deadlines and targets to meet, customers to keep happy, etc. Although he likes the fact that modern technology has made communication with customers so much faster, he feels that it adds a great deal to his workload — i.e. he now has messages to reply to on his e-mail, fax and mobile phone as well as taking telephone calls and replying to mail queries. Because of this increase in workload he normally rushes lunch by eating fast food or a sandwich with a soft drink or more coffee. Afternoons are hectic as he is out visiting clients and the traffic in Dublin can be hellish. When he comes home in the evenings he is always tense and frustrated, and there are always bits of unfinished work. He eats his main meal of the day around eight-thirty or nine o'clock while watching television.

Stress can be helpful in that it gets us up and active and doing hopefully meaningful things with our lives; however, too much stress can have a negative effect on our well-being. As one reformed alcoholic once told me (reformed alcoholics are some of the wisest people that I have met), there are twenty-four hours in the day and balanced human beings spend eight of them sleeping, eight of them working and eight of them relaxing. This is easy to say but hard to stick to, especially if you have responsibilities to meet — bills to pay, children to look after, etc. When stress starts to have a negative effect, the digestive system is the first to suffer. Firstly, we tend to disregard the quality of the food we are eating; convenience and fast foods are more acceptable because we often do not have enough time to eat. Secondly, we tend to eat when we are tense and anxious; also, we eat while preoccupied with our work. Thirdly, we tend to eat the main meal too late in the day, when the body is preparing for a night's rest. Fourthly, we tend to use stimulants — tea, coffee, caffeine — to perk us up, and relaxants such as alcohol to calm us down. This wreaks havoc with the nervous system, but because we get caught in a vicious cycle we find it hard to stop.

STRESS AND EATING HABITS

Let's now analyse John's diet and eating habits. Firstly, let's look at his eating habits. He eats nothing for breakfast, then has coffee early in the morning, followed by more coffee with refined foods (muffins and biscuits) later in the morning. This is then followed by a light lunch of more refined carbohydrates (fast foods and white bread) with more coffee or a soft drink. The main meal is then eaten late at night.

The times at which you eat are extremely important. The wise old saying: 'Eat breakfast like a prince, eat lunch like a king and eat supper like a pauper' is worth remembering. Eat when your digestion is most efficient, i.e. between 10 a.m. and 3 p.m. approximately. This is when you are mentally and physically most efficient. Do not put a heavy workload on the digestive system when it is preparing to rest, i.e. at night; if you do, food will just sit there undigested and it will ferment or putrefy. You can get away with doing this occasionally, but if done frequently you will induce chronic digestive problems.

There is another wise saying relating to digestion: 'After dinner rest a while, after supper walk a mile.' My mother used to say this all the time.

In her day, the main meal was in the middle of the day and was then called dinner. Because a lot of energy is needed to digest food, it is best to rest after a heavy meal. This allows for a good blood supply to the digestive tract. When I was a child, supper was a very light meal, e.g. tea and toast. In this way we went to bed with little food in our stomachs and woke up hungry in the morning. You will find that people who eat late at night eat little or nothing in the mornings as they will not be hungry; indeed food may irritate the lining of the digestive tract for such people. If you do have to eat a substantial meal after 5 p.m., make sure to exercise — go for a brisk walk to get the digestive system back into action to ensure that the food is digested efficiently. All of these old sayings make a lot of sense; they were passed down from generation to generation for a good reason.

What about eating when tense or anxious or frustrated? Many of us have to eat on the run these days because our lives are so hectic. We also eat without taking time to unwind and relax. Remember that the French and some other Europeans take three hours off in the middle of the day to have lunch. They begin with an aperitif (e.g. anise) to stimulate the secretion of digestive juices and to act as a relaxant. Time is taken to taste and appreciate the food, and then, after eating, time is taken to relax, socialise and digest the food. This is the ideal way to eat. At least take one hour to have lunch and make it a substantial meal. Do not engage in work-related activities or anything that might make you tense, e.g. watching television, reading newspapers, etc. Eat only what pleases you and chew it well; do not eat only what is convenient. Eat with people whose company you enjoy and relax for a while afterwards.

When stressed we often adopt sloppy eating habits and ignore what is good for us. We eat lots of refined foods and ignore nutritious foods such as fruit, vegetables, etc. Ensure that what you eat is adequately absorbed by relaxing afterwards; remember that the food you consume is the nourishment for the rest of your body and that it will never get to the rest of your body, regardless of how nutritious it is, if it is not absorbed efficiently. So, allow your tummy time and space to do its work. If you are under pressure of time, eat something that is easy to digest (e.g. soup), or eat nothing at all.

STRESS AND DIET
Have you noticed that when people become stressed or emotionally upset they find it much harder to stick to a diet or to an exercise programme. They tend to abandon good foods, e.g. wholegrains, for refined convenience foods. Let's look at John's diet in more detail and see how healthy it is. He has coffee as soon as he arrives at work and then later on again. It is very typical of a stressed person to use strong stimulants such as coffee to boost their energy levels. Stress depletes the body of energy and so stimulants like coffee, tea, caffeine and sugar are used to give you a quick lift. If you need an energy boost it would be much safer to use a good B complex vitamin supplement along with Panax ginseng, for example. Keep some at work if you have a stressful job and use them to help you through the day. They are not addictive and will help your body cope better with stress.

Convenience foods, especially those made from refined carbohydrates — white flour and white sugar — such as muffins, cakes, pies, pizza, biscuits, hot dogs and hamburger rolls, are used by people who are very busy and want something to fill a hole in their stomachs. Too much refined carbohydrates, like stimulants, can also upset the hormonal system and the nervous system. The ups and downs in the blood sugar level that occur when refined carbohydrates are consumed disturb the body. They put stress on the pancreas to produce more insulin, and on the adrenal glands to produce cortisol and adrenaline. This can cause the blood sugar level to drop below normal (hypoglycaemia). Eating sugary foods occasionally does not cause too much difficulty — it is only when the pancreas and adrenal glands are constantly stressed that problems such as hypoglycaemia arise.

In summary then, John's diet is too high in stimulants and refined carbohydrates. Try to use what nature provides, e.g. get your sugar from the fructose in fruit, honey and dried fruit, and use wholegrain cereals and breads. These will nourish you and stabilise your blood sugar levels and so you will have better energy levels.

EFFECTS OF STRESS ON THE DIGESTIVE SYSTEM

Stress affects all parts of the digestive tract, from mouth to anus. Before examining how stress affects each individual part of the digestive tract, let's see how it affects the nervous system, which controls the digestive process.

Figure 4.1 *EFFECTS OF STRESS ON DIGESTION*

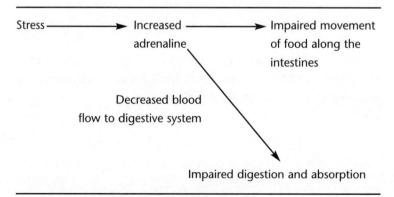

The pulse, blood pressure, breathing and peristalsis (rhythmic contractions of the intestinal wall) are all controlled by the involuntary nervous system. We do not control these bodily functions consciously; rather they happen naturally. However, any disruption to the involuntary nervous system can have far-reaching effects. For example, when we are stressed or anxious, the adrenal glands pump out adrenaline, which is one of the hormones that affect the involuntary nervous system. Adrenaline will increase your heart rate and blood pressure, but will decrease peristalsis, thereby slowing the movement of food along the intestines. Adrenaline will also shift blood away from the intestinal wall, thereby slowing digestion of food and absorption. Hence the feeling of nausea and butterflies when acutely stressed. If the stress is prolonged, digestion will be chronically upset, and therefore food will end up being incompletely digested and may ferment and putrefy.

The involuntary nervous system is under the control of hormones such as adrenaline. Too much adrenaline can cause ongoing digestive problems. For example, many conventional doctors have seen a very strong link between irritable bowel syndrome and stress. Many clinical studies have verified this link.

Now you can see how hormones interact very closely with the nervous system — so much so that the two systems are now taught in medical school as one system, the neuro-endocrine system.

Figure 4.2 gives an overview of how stress affects different parts of the digestive tract. Let's look at the effects of ongoing stress on each part individually.

Figure 4.2 *EFFECTS OF STRESS ON THE DIGESTIVE TRACT*

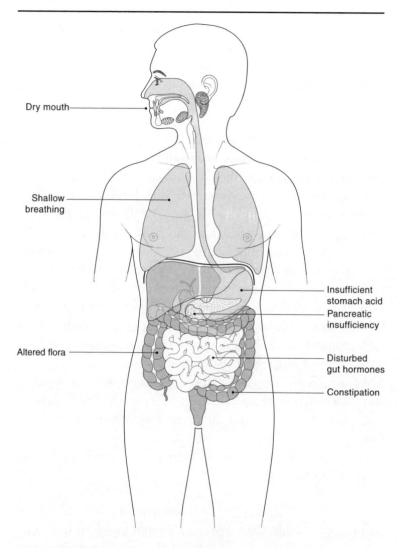

Dry mouth

Shallow breathing

Altered flora

Insufficient stomach acid

Pancreatic insufficiency

Disturbed gut hormones

Constipation

THE EFFECTS ON THE PRODUCTION OF SALIVA

Saliva, as you have already learned, contains an enzyme called salivary amylase, which digests carbohydrates (starch and sugars). So, carbohydrate digestion actually begins in the mouth. Stress reduces the amount of saliva produced by the salivary glands; hence, it impairs carbohydrate digestion.

Saliva also softens and moistens food, making it easier to swallow. Have you noticed how dry your mouth can become when you are acutely stressed? If there is ongoing stress it makes it very difficult to swallow food.

Stress therefore has a negative effect on the digestion and swallowing of food.

THE EFFECTS ON THE PRODUCTION OF STOMACH ACID

Chronic stress suppresses stomach acid production. The symptoms associated with low stomach acid are exactly the same as the symptoms associated with high stomach acid. These symptoms include a feeling of fullness, discomfort, burping, bad breath, flatulence and pain. As the two conditions are hard to distinguish, the only way to diagnose them is by taking some stomach acid (betaine hydrochloride) in tablet form, and if the symptoms improve then low stomach acid can be diagnosed. Failure to improve after taking a betaine hydrochloride tablet would suggest a condition of high stomach acid. This is the simplest and least interventional way of separating the two conditions.

As low stomach acid may also be associated with zinc deficiency — the production of stomach acid is dependent on zinc — use about 20 mg of chelated zinc daily with food.

Obviously, the best way to treat low stomach acid is to treat the underlying stress.

THE EFFECTS ON BREATHING

Breathing is something that you do not think about consciously; it is under the control of the involuntary nervous system. (I refer to this part of the nervous system as the adrenaline/noradrenaline system, since adrenaline speeds you up and noradrenaline calms you down. One's day is supposed to be balanced by periods of activity — adrenaline release — and periods of rest and relaxation — noradrenaline release.

Too much adrenaline or noradrenaline leads to an imbalance in the involuntary nervous system, causing problems with the sweat glands, heart rate, rate and depth of breathing). During periods of stress, your rate and depth of breathing changes. Because of a higher output of adrenaline in stressful situations, your breathing tends to be much faster and shallower. Because of the shallow breathing, you have to take a deep breath occasionally to get more oxygen into the bloodstream. People under stress can cope much better if they learn to control their breathing, ensuring that they take deep breaths. For example, I find that many people with high blood pressure can drop their blood pressure merely by taking three deep breaths. Try it sometime for yourself.

Now look at Figure 4.3.

There is a sheet of muscle called the diaphragm which separates the chest from the abdomen. When you breathe in, the diaphragm moves downwards and flattens out, thereby increasing the space in the chest cavity so that your lungs can expand. On exhaling, the diaphragm moves upwards and pushes air out of the lungs. This rhythmic motion of the diaphragm has the effect of massaging the digestive organs, thereby improving their function. Because you do not breathe deeply when stressed the diaphragm does not descend much and so does not stimulate the digestive tract in the same way.

So, stress has a negative effect not only on your rate and depth of breathing but also has a negative knock-on effect on the digestive system.

THE EFFECTS ON THE PANCREAS

The pancreas is often called the stress organ of the body because it is here that the effects of stress are most pronounced. Stress disrupts the production of insulin and the production of digestive juices — the two major functions of the pancreas. Both of these functions are under the control of the neuro-endocrine system.

Figure 4.3 *DIAPHRAGM SEPARATES THE THORAX FROM THE ABDOMEN*

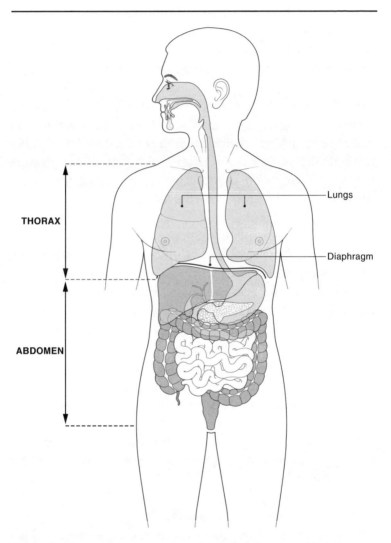

Stress leads to an increase in adrenaline levels, which in turn causes an increase in the blood sugar level. The pancreas responds to this rise in blood sugar level by releasing more insulin — this shifts the sugar out of the bloodstream and into the cells for the release of energy. When the stress is prolonged, the pancreas finds it more and more difficult to respond quickly and so the blood sugar level becomes more difficult to control. The pancreas becomes depleted.

The other main job of the pancreas is to produce digestive juices. The secretion of these juices is under the control of a hormone called secretin.

Secretin is released from the wall of the duodenum as soon as food begins to leave the stomach. This hormone is part of a number of hormones that control the whole digestive tract. All of these hormones are under the control of the involuntary nervous system. When stress acts via the involuntary nervous system, it causes a decrease in the release of secretin, and hence less digestive juice will be secreted by the pancreas.

So, stress has a double effect on the pancreas — by changing its capacity to respond to blood sugar level, as well as reducing its digestive capacity. This latter effect impairs the digestion of all food groups, i.e. carbohydrates, fats and proteins.

Figure 4.4 *EFFECTS OF STRESS ON THE PANCREAS*

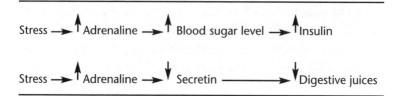

EFFECTS ON THE MICROFLORA

A healthy bacterial environment in the digestive tract is essential for your state of health — these bacteria form the first line of defence against pathogens and so protect against intestinal infections. The intestinal flora also protect against bowel cancer and assist the absorption of calcium across the intestinal wall. Prolonged periods of stress upset the bacterial flora, allowing bad bacteria, yeast and fungi to thrive.

This affects your immunity as well as your vitamin status — good bacteria manufacture a number of B vitamins as well as vitamin K, all of which are absorbed across the intestinal wall. So, good bacteria not only feed us with vitamins but protect us from infection.

Anyone who has suffered from a prolonged period of stress should take a good multi-vitamin supplement as well as a probiotic containing the 'good' bacteria, such as acidophilus and bifidus; these are available at any healthfood shop.

EFFECTS ON THE HORMONAL SYSTEM

The secretion of the digestive juices by the stomach and small intestine is under hormonal control. For example, the sight, smell or taste of food sends a message via the nervous system to the brain, which then relays a message to the stomach to secrete a hormone called gastrin. This hormone controls the secretion of gastric juices. Low levels of gastrin will result in small amounts of gastric juice being secreted.

The release of food from the stomach into the small intestine stimulates the release of another hormone called secretin, which controls the release of digestive enzymes from the pancreas. In fact, the whole of the digestive process is under the control of the hormonal system. The release of these hormones is in turn under the control of the nervous system. This is illustrated in Figure 4.5 below.

Figure 4.5 *THE ROLE OF HORMONES IN DIGESTION*

Sight/smell/ ⟶ Brain ⟶ Involuntary ⟶ Release ⟶ Secretion
taste of   nervous   of the   of digestive
food   sytem   hormone   juices
                                       gastrin

We have learned that chronic stress acts via the involuntary nervous system to disturb hormonal levels in the digestive tract. Figure 4.6 shows how a disturbance in the hormonal levels will also affect the secretion of digestive juices all the along the digestive tract. The lower the level of hormone, the less the amount of juice secreted. When this happens, food cannot be digested efficiently or completely. Food therefore ends up being partly digested or undigested. This food then becomes highly toxic as it ferments or putrefies, producing nasty chemicals that inflame the intestinal wall. This is why the abdomen can be quite tender to press on.

Hence, stress disturbs the digestive process very significantly.

Figure 4.6 *EFFECTS OF STRESS ON HORMONES AND DIGESTION*

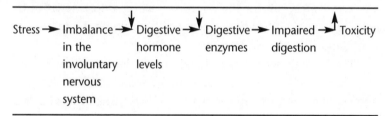

Stress also affects the blood supply to the small intestine. It causes the release of adrenaline, which increases the blood flow to the muscles — to get you ready for action — at the expense of the digestive tract. This means that both digestion and absorption of food can be impaired. In order to function correctly, the cells of the digestive tract, like cells anywhere else in the body, need nourishment and oxygen supplied by the bloodstream. If this blood supply is reduced, neither food nor oxygen can be supplied in optimal amounts; hence these cells lining the digestive tract cannot secrete optimal levels of the enzymes and fluid needed for digestion.

Again, the food ends up being incompletely digested and then becoming highly toxic. If these toxins cross the intestinal wall into the bloodstream, they can end up causing symptoms elsewhere in the body. (I shall discuss these symptoms in Chapter 6.)

As you can see, stress has far-reaching effects; the initial effects are felt in the digestive tract but, if prolonged, all systems of the body can become affected. Ultimately, one's mental and emotional well-being is affected also. Therefore, never underestimate the effects of stress on your health.

CASE HISTORY — SHEILA: IRRITABLE BOWEL SYNDROME (IBS)

Sheila had been diagnosed by her GP as having irritable bowel syndrome (IBS). She had been referred to a gastro-enterologist for tests, all of which proved to be negative. Because her symptoms were suggestive of IBS, her GP decided to treat it as such, with conventional drugs — anti-spasmodics for the pain and anti-diarrhoeals for the diarrhoea, along with a sedative to help her anxiety. After six months on these drugs she felt much worse and sought help from me.

When I tested her she had significant gut fermentation, in fact it was the worst case I have seen so far; however, she also had significant emotional stress in her life — her husband was having an affair.

I began by dealing with the digestive problem, and then referred her to a family counsellor for help with her marital problem. Two months later there were definite signs of improvement — she was off all conventional treatment, had no further episodes of pain and her bowel habit had improved. What pleased her most was the fact that her husband was co-operating in having joint counselling.

Often IBS is diagnosed when doctors and practitioners do not know what is wrong. It is diagnosed when all the conventional tests prove negative and when the person experiences pain and diarrhoea, with or without mucus in the stool. If you have such symptoms, seek help and try to identify the cause. In my experience IBS is often caused by dysbiosis or by fermentation. Both of these conditions take time to heal but are eminently treatable.

CASE HISTORY — ELLEN: PEPTIC ULCER

Ellen was a very attractive sixty-year-old lady who had two sons who were very dependent on her. She was a very wealthy woman, having been left a lot of money by her husband, who died five years previously. Ellen complained of severe abdominal pain after eating, associated with nausea, and on occasion had vomited. Sometimes she had to get up at night to relieve the symptoms with warm milk and biscuits.

I made a provisional diagnosis of peptic ulcer and referred her for a blood test, which confirmed the presence of *Helicobacter pylori*, the bacteria that is associated with peptic ulcers. I treated her using herbal remedies and asked her to adjust her lifestyle by taking regular exercise, avoiding stimulants, sugar, alcohol and spicy foods, and to discuss the stress in her life with a stress counsellor — she was under constant pressure as her two sons were very dependent on her and very demanding.

She did not respond well to the physical treatment initially, and it was only when she started to manage her personal relationship with her sons that she showed improvement. This is often the case when there is ongoing stress in one's life, i.e. the physical symptoms only show improvement once the stress is under control.

CASE HISTORY — JOHN: PAIN IN THE ANAL SPHINCTER

John worked abroad in the stock exchange and was back home in Ireland for a short visit. He came to see me complaining of tightness and pain in the anal sphincter, which made it difficult to have a bowel motion. This problem was getting worse and he was very worried about it. John had noticed that the condition disappeared when he was on holidays. More recently, he had been getting short bouts of palpitations lasting only a minute or two intermittently. He described his job as very stressful, as he had to do many things at the same time. He also had to travel a considerable distance to and from his workplace and was essentially away from home for thirteen hours a day.

I treated John by giving him relaxation exercises to do every day. I prescribed ginseng and vitamin B complex and asked him to take up yoga or meditation. He improved a lot physically, but more importantly he became aware of what his stressful lifestyle was doing to him and is now seeking a new job. He also became aware of other aspects of his lifestyle, in particular his eating habits and the importance of having sufficient energy to enjoy time with his family.

A wonderful change took place in this man. Stress can have a positive value — it can drive you to make meaningful changes in your life.

Summary

Negative stress can make life very difficult. We often abandon regular eating habits and a good diet, and we often stop exercising.

Stress usually first manifests as physical symptoms in the digestive tract — stomach pain, change in bowel habit, gurgling, flatulence and bloating. Later, energy levels tend to fluctuate as both the digestion and the absorption of food become impaired. Our breathing can also become shallow as a consequence of stress.

It is important to not only treat the physical symptoms but also to seek help through stress management or counselling.

5

EMOTIONAL PROBLEMS

Let me illustrate how emotional problems can be at the root of physical problems by giving you the following example. James is a well-dressed businessman, who is a perfectionist. He demands high standards from himself and all who work for him. He works long hours and often does not understand when others cannot. He is irritable and edgy a lot of the time. His business is booming but his body is not. He has significant digestive problems, including a duodenal ulcer, abdominal bloating, flatulence and very loose stools, with blood and mucus in the stool on occasion. Because he is not in pain he does not seek help for these complaints.

James often goes to his local golf club for a few drinks after work, but he has found that he cannot tolerate alcohol that well of late. In the mornings he always wakes up feeling groggy and hungover, even though he drinks lots of water before bedtime. His wife is fed up listening to him complaining about his tummy and has given up telling him to go to the doctor.

One night James woke up with a pain in his stomach so severe that he asked his wife to call for an ambulance. In hospital he was diagnosed as having a perforated ulcer and was prepared for an emergency operation. He recovered well following the operation but was very shaken by the whole experience. He was aware that he had come close to death.

Thereafter James paid more attention to his physical symptoms and came to me to help solve his ongoing tummy problems, i.e. the bloating, wind and loose stools.

On taking a detailed history from James, it became clear that he had a lot of repressed anger. He had developed the habit of not expressing his anger — a habit that went back to his childhood, because his father had been very abusive and James had been scared of him; it was safer for James not to express his emotions and so he learned to suppress them. Any time he got angry as an adult he would stay quiet, push himself that bit harder at work and overindulge in alcohol and rich food; that was his way of coping. However, emotions like anger will express themselves by one means or another; in other words, if you do not express the anger it will upset the physical body, creating physical symptoms and ultimately causing you damage. James was beginning to understand this concept.

I suggested that he buy himself a punch-bag and a pair of boxing gloves and beat the hell out of the bag anytime he felt a surge of anger or anytime he felt frustrated. I also suggested that he take up one of the martial arts, both for exercise and for venting aggression in a constructive way.

I performed a number of investigations on James to find out the state of his digestive tract. I discovered that he had a number of problems. He was not digesting his food properly, the bacterial population was grossly abnormal and he had parasites. After three months of treatment James began to show improvement. He was slow to improve initially, as he had found it hard to alter his lifestyle — changes included diet, exercise, no alcohol on social and business occasions, and taking medicines. He no longer had any digestive complaints and his stool was more solid and normal. His energy and sense of well-being had improved remarkably. Even his relationship with his wife had improved, as he was able to speak about his difficulties more openly.

James's case is an excellent example of how emotions can interact with the physical body — the digestive tract in this case. Suppression of emotions such as anger can underlie many digestive complaints such as gastritis, ulcers, gut fermentation, pancreatic problems. Fear and anger are two energetic disturbances that can wreak havoc in the digestive tract. When you are frightened you get butterflies in your stomach; if the fear continues and becomes chronic the digestive disturbances can be significant. In the West there is an epidemic of digestive problems as the pressures on people — time pressures, financial pressures, etc. — increase; since Western civilisation is driven by fear and anger, this is hardly surprising.

THE SOLAR PLEXUS

The belief that digestive problems arise from disturbances in our emotions is far from new. This fact has been recognised for centuries by almost every culture. At an emotional level, when you feel angry, frustrated or upset about some particular event in your life, e.g. a break-up with a loved one, we say that you have difficulty 'stomaching' what has happened; many languages have sayings indicating this connection between one's feelings and one's digestion. The 'solar plexus', which is the seat of our deeper feelings, is located in the abdomen. In our everyday lives we know that the workings of the digestive tract are sensitive to our emotional state.

Until recently, conventional medicine believed that the emotional centre in the body was located in the brain only. There has now been a revolution in neuroscience: it has been discovered that all the neurotransmitters that control brain activity are also located in the gut. It has also been discovered that the brain and the gut can communicate with one another and so influence each other. We are now beginning to understand how our emotions are expressed in the digestive tract.

For example, it is known that all drugs that act on the central nervous system have gastrointestinal side effects; Prozac not only acts on serotonin levels in the brain but also affects serotonin levels in the gut. The same is true of painkillers, sedatives, anti-anxiety drugs and antidepressants.

It is also now known that people with digestive problems such as fermentation can have sleep disturbances as well. Scientists know that sleep is composed of ninety-minute cycles of slow brainwave sleep, followed by periods of REM (rapid eye movement) sleep. The gut nervous system works in synchronicity with this pattern and produces a ninety-minute cycle of slow wave muscle contractions, followed by periods of rapid muscle contraction. The two nervous systems work in harmony and communicate with one another via the release of neurotransmitters. Hence, anything that upsets the release of neurotransmitters in one system has a direct effect on the other system. These discoveries are fascinating and indicate the connectedness of all bodily functions.

We tend to think of the immune system as white blood cells circulating in the bloodstream. The truth, however, is that the major part of the immune system resides in the digestive tract. In addition to the billions of bacteria — the 'flora' — that protect the whole length of the digestive tract by acting like soldiers, the gut wall also has large patches of lymphoid tissue that manufacture lymphocytes to fight off invaders. This lymphoid tissue is referred to as *gut-associated lymphatic tissue* (GALT). This tissue responds to any invader or foreign substance in the same way that the tonsils do, and, like the tonsils, this tissue can become inflamed and swollen. Children who react to the measles virus or to oral polio drops given as vaccinations early in childhood may end up with chronic inflammation in the gut. Researchers at the Royal Free Hospital in London are suggesting that a reaction to the MMR vaccine in particular may cause inflammatory bowel disease later in life.

All in all, the gut is a very sophisticated and complex system. It has a brain of its own — nerves, neurotransmitters, sensory tissue — as well as a well-equipped army of bacteria and a large amount of lymphoid tissue, the GALT. As a result, your emotions are not only reflected in your digestion but also in your immune status.

Emotional stress can cause infections.

CASE HISTORY — MARY: RECURRENT INFECTIONS

Mary came to me for help as she was constantly getting what she called bouts of glandular fever. She had been getting these bouts of fever, with swollen glands, sore throat and aches and pains, for over two years and had failed to find a cause. All of her medical tests were negative, except that her lymphocyte count was increased, suggesting a viral infection. I therefore asked her if anything traumatic, especially of an emotional nature, had happened within the previous three years. She told me that she had lost her father and her husband in a car accident three years previously, and because she had two small children she had to 'keep going' for their sake. She had never really taken the time to grieve properly because of the constant demands of daily life and having to cope with young children. She was desperately trying to cope, but her body was clearly not co-operating; it was indicating that there was a problem, and a deep-seated one at that.

I suggested that she go to a counsellor for help and, since I knew one who was a true healer, I referred her there. I also prescribed an immune-boosting herbal medicine and did not see her again until eight months later. She told me how relieved she felt — it was as if someone had lifted a great weight from her shoulders; she was able to let her husband and father go in an emotional sense and was able to speak more easily about how she felt. This had a wonderful knock-on effect on her children, who also sensed that they could release their feelings about the deaths as well. Interestingly, her physical health had improved and she no longer experiences bouts of illness.

Suppressing one's emotions does not work; emotions need expression and have the power to cause physical difficulties until they eventually find expression.

Mary had a remarkably strong constitution and handled the loss of two very important people in her life with enormous courage and strength. It was a testimony to her own inner strength that she did not end up with a more serious illness. She got rid of her viral illness and regained full health.

FEAR

The biggest barrier to people achieving their full potential as human beings is *fear*. The biggest block preventing someone from healing fully is *fear*.

Fear is part of the human condition, and the game of life is about conquering it. It has the power to cripple you and reduce you to total inactivity or you can face your fear and fight to conquer it. Most people who have had to face their fears will tell you that the thought of facing it is worse than actually facing it. Often facing our fears has a powerful liberating effect and allows us to follow our true path in life fearlessly. But before we can find our true destiny or pathway in life, it is necessary to be challenged by having to face our greatest fear; this is often referred to as the 'dark night of the soul'. Many years ago a very wise man told me that one's greatest nightmare is one's wildest dream trying to come true. I didn't understand what he meant at the time and it has taken me many years to really understand the truth of this saying; it means that one has to face one's greatest fear before one's wildest dream can come true.

We all fear something in life; many of our fears are irrational and we cannot explain why we are so afraid of spiders, heights, etc. Some fears can have deep-seated effects on our physical and mental well-being, for example people who have been raped are often afraid of losing control of their environment and will expend endless energy trying desperately to control it.

Fear resides in the digestive tract and leads to chronic disturbances. It is relatively easy to correct these disturbances in the physical body, but it is a lot harder to diminish the fear in someone; hence my earlier statement about fear being a big block in the healing process. However, if the digestive disturbances are to disappear permanently, the fear must be confronted and dealt with, thereby freeing the person to appreciate the beauty of life.

Irritable bowel syndrome is a good example of how deep-seated fears can upset the digestive tract on an ongoing basis.

CASE HISTORY — JANET: IRRITABLE BOWEL SYNDROME (IBS)

Janet worked in the Middle East as a nurse and was sent home because she was having ongoing bowel problems. After many medical investigations it was found that she had parasites, but despite treatment she did not improve. Her doctor then diagnosed her with IBS and said that there was nothing further he could do. She therefore sought help from alternative medicine rather reluctantly and came to see me.

What became clear from talking to her was her skilful avoidance in answering questions relating to her feelings. She did not wish to talk about her emotional state and so I respected her wishes and began physical treatment to assist her digestion. I saw her frequently initially so that she got used to me, and I was hoping at some point she would feel it was safe to confide in me. Two months later, after she had interrogated me sufficiently, she decided to open up and told me that she had been raped repeatedly by her uncle when she was quite young. Her uncle had died recently and she was now having nightmares about him; she felt his presence in her bedroom on many occasions. This explained much about Janet — her need to test me first before confiding in me, her need to control everything in her life, her failure to have a normal relationship with a man.

I used hypnosis to help her access some of the anger and fear which were the controlling influences in her life. It is only by bringing these to the conscious level that we become aware of the effect they are having on us; when they are left hidden in the subconscious mind they can wreak havoc in a person's life, because only the effects can be seen and never the cause. It is by bringing them to the conscious awareness of the person that they can be diminished and so have less control over the person.

I later referred Janet to a counsellor to help her become more aware of her feelings and to express them in some way — verbally, through dance, music, art, etc. Until her emotional health improved it was not possible to speak of a permanent solution to her digestive problem.

Today she has made enormous progress and is presently helping rape victims as a counsellor. She is acutely aware now of the connection between her emotional state and digestion — when she gets upset or frustrated she immediately gets an upset tummy. When she sees these warning signs she expresses her feelings to her partner and so is able to prevent a recurrence of the IBS.

I find it interesting that when people who have experienced great difficulties in their lives, such as rape, heal themselves, they will often end up helping those with similar difficulties.

EXPRESSING EMOTIONS

In the Western world we are physically and mentally very active, running around chasing our tails with our heads full of things to remember to do. We seldom take the time to be quiet, to reflect and to express our deepest emotions. We have little time to feel, to listen to what our heart is saying and to express what is so critical for our well-being to express. Functioning on a physical and mental level and blocking our emotions is a more comfortable and convenient way to exist. However, life is about love, not convenience and comfort and 'success' in material terms. How can we express the love in our hearts if we are consumed with fear, anger, hatred?

We will never understand the essence of life as long as we are driven by fear or anger. To become whole again we have to begin by acknowledging the fear or anger within; then we have to confront this fear or anger and see clearly the negative effect these emotions can have on our own well-being and that of our loved ones, and ultimately on society as a whole; finally, we have to then express this fear or anger via words, music, art, sculpture, dance, etc. — one of the more constructive ways to express anger is to beat the hell out of a punch-bag. Self-development courses can be enormously helpful in making you aware of the emotional energy that drives you. Hypnosis is also extraordinarily helpful. Personally, I was never aware of how critical I was of myself and therefore of others until I had a few sessions of hypnosis; I was alarmed at how severely criticised I was as a child at school and what a deep impact it had on my whole life thereafter. This subconscious information is like gold dust, as it allows you to see what is driving you, and then, if you choose to do so, free yourself from it.

To block your emotions is to block your very essence; you suffocate your true self and your true potential. By doing so you have an unseen negative effect on the lives of others. People are uplifted by a free, loving, innocent person and pulled down by a false, fearful, angry, unloving person. Your energy interacts with and affects everyone around you. Become aware, acknowledge the truth of who you are at this point in time by bringing what is in the subconscious to the surface for you to see it, and if you want to change seek help.

The truth is that we have all grown up in a very negative era and we are all wounded in some way. We have all inherited fear and anger from our parents, teachers, clergy, etc., and these emotions are slowly destroying individuals via alcohol and drugs; they are also, in more subtle ways, destroying our society. Blocked emotion, especially blocked anger, is a very destructive force.

You may now appreciate my need to establish a healing centre where people not only get physical help but also have the chance to transform themselves in a very positive way by unblocking negative emotions. Healing is really, in essence, a process of unblocking.

If you are to heal, as distinct from treat, your digestive problem, you have to explore your emotions — acknowledge, confront and express your emotions!

Everyone that I treat has an emotional component to their illness to a greater or lesser extent. Most are not ready to acknowledge it and so come for treatment; it is only when they are ready that they will heal. The next case history is a simple example of blocked anger causing a digestive disturbance.

CASE HISTORY — BRENDA: PANCREATITIS

Brenda had suffered from bowel problems continuously for eight years and was getting worse to the point where she was becoming intolerant to many of the foods that had previously formed the bulk of her diet. After eating wheat, dairy produce, sugar, yeast foods and potatoes, she developed abdominal bloating, loose, pale and offensive stools, flatulence and a significant drop in her energy level. She also suffered from hypoglycaemia on occasions, and cold hands and feet most of the time.

After extensive tests I diagnosed her as having pancreatitis, a not uncommon condition but one that is seldom diagnosed. I treated her using diet, nutritional supplements and homeopathy. I was also aware that chronic pancreatitis is often associated with emotional stress, so we discussed the stresses in her life. To cut a long story short, she had tremendous anger directed against her father, who was an alcoholic and had abandoned the family when Brenda was nine years old. She had a tremendous sense of not only anger but abandonment and had a great distrust of men. Since the upper abdomen is an emotional zone in the body, deeply felt emotions such as anger can manifest in this region.

Since Brenda was consciously aware of the emotional source of her difficulty and did not need help with bringing it to the surface, as so many of us do, I referred her to a wonderful healer who did a technique called Somato-Emotional Release, which is really unlocking emotional energy blocks in the physical body (the soma). Today Brenda is indeed a transformed person who is not just physically well and able to tolerate a normal diet but emotionally very strong too. In Brenda's case it was necessary to provide both physical and emotional treatment simultaneously to gain such improvement.

How Our Emotions Affect Digestion

It should be appreciated that the abdomen is the main centre of our physical nourishment, but also tied into that is our emotional nourishment. It dates back to the time that we are in the womb, when we are connected to our mother's body via the umbilical cord. This cord supplies food and oxygen directly from our mother's body. We can say that we are physically attached but we are also emotionally attached. It is now known that the emotions of the mother are reflected in the baby's body.

In young children it is very common to find that they complain of a sore tummy when they are emotionally upset. When asked to show where it hurts they will inevitably point to their umbilicus. It is clear that emotions are linked to our abdomen and in particular to the digestive tract and its appendages such as the pancreas and the liver.

Science now agrees with this, since it has been discovered that all the neurotransmitters in the brain are also in the digestive tract. These neurotransmitters are the means by which our emotional state is expressed. For example, a positive emotional state is reflected in the levels of these neurotransmitters as a balance or homeostasis; a negative emotional state creates an imbalance in the level of neuro-transmitters. Similarly, anything that disturbs the neuro-transmitter levels, e.g. drugs such as Prozac, cocaine, alcohol, will also affect one's emotional state. Since these neuro-transmitters control the digestive system it is not hard to see how the emotional state and the digestive process interact with one another; one is reflected in the other.

With anger and fear being so prevalent in people in the Western world, it is not hard to see why digestive problems are so common. This is why my teacher of natural medicine used to say that one should never eat when emotionally upset and one should never eat reading mail or watching television or reading the newspaper, as all of these activities can upset us emotionally. Eat in a quiet, relaxed environment.

Lack of awareness about how digestion interacts with our emotional state can lead to chronic digestive problems and, if left untreated, cancer. I have read many authoritative books on bowel cancer but none of them mentioned suppressed emotions as a causative factor. I personally believe that this is the most important cause. The next case history illustrates the point well.

Case History — Frank: Bowel Cancer

Frank had suffered from chronic constipation for most of his life and then at the age of fifty was diagnosed with colon cancer. He was combining what alternative and conventional medicine had to offer in an attempt to treat the cancer. I was guiding him about the best forms of treatment available in natural medicine. One day he came to see me because he was very distraught at what had happened at home. He was very angry at something his young son had done and had beaten him so hard it had actually upset him emotionally. Frank was aware that he could die from cancer and lived with this reality. He loved his children and had got much closer to them since the diagnosis of cancer. This sudden venting of anger had alarmed him and he came to me quite upset about it as he did not want to hurt his children.

I spent some time exploring Frank's own life, especially his childhood, and learned that he harboured a lot of anger against the Christian Brothers who had taught him at school. He had been beaten almost daily at school because he had been dyslexic. He was also beaten at home by his father on occasion, but he felt that most of those beatings had some justification; the ones at school had no justification and so he was very resentful and angry — as a child he had been very anxious and frightened about going to school. He had buried these feelings for years. It was only when he was faced with cancer that he sought help and so was more open to healing all aspects of himself, including his emotions. I explained to him that when you open yourself to healing, emotions from the past that have been buried can surface out of the blue and must be released; however, they must be released in a constructive way. Hurting his son had a very negative effect on Frank, but when I explained that releasing suppressed anger is very positive he felt better. I asked him to apologise to his son and explain to him what had happened. Children are enormously understanding and forgiving. I suggested that he vent his anger by going into the woods and screaming, or by punching a punch-bag or by taking up one of the martial arts. He took my advice and bought a punch-bag. He has taught his son to release his anger in a constructive way also.

Children often reflect where the parent/s are at emotionally. As in Frank's case, it is important to teach them how to heal by example so that if they experience difficulties in their own lives they will have had a good role model and will know what to do.

CASE HISTORY — MICHELLE: CHRONIC DIARRHOEA

Michelle came to me to help her solve an ongoing digestive problem. She had chronic diarrhoea and was beginning to lose weight; she also complained of bloating and gurgling sounds from her tummy. More recently she was also experiencing loss of appetite as she had constant nausea. Michelle was only twenty-nine years old and yet had a whole litany of digestive complaints. She was very unpopular with my reception staff as she was aggressive in her dealings with people. It was also noticeable in the consulting room; it was as if she had a high-voltage electric fence around her that could fire sparks in my direction with the slightest provocation. She employed this aggression in her work, as she worked for the debt collection department of a major financial institution.

I invited Michelle to come to a weekend workshop that I was running; I felt that she would benefit from it as it was about self-awareness. She attended, but little did she know that she would spend most of the weekend in tears, and at one point her whole body began to tremble uncontrollably. We were doing a relaxation exercise and the instructor was teaching us self-hypnosis and took us into a state of hypnosis; it was at this point that all her pain started to surface and continued to surface for the whole weekend. She had suffered a lot of physical and sexual abuse growing up and ended up being a very angry and aggressive woman. After the weekend, which she found very helpful as it opened her eyes to what had for so long been hidden beneath the surface, she went for counselling, for hypnosis and for help from the Rape Crisis Centre. It took time for her digestive system to improve because she went through a tough time emotionally, but improve it did. She became acutely aware of the connection between her emotional state and her digestion, as any emotional crisis led to a sudden deterioration in her digestive system. It was only when she gained emotional stability again that her nausea disappeared to the point where she felt hungry again, and she began to regain lost weight. She left her job and did a course in counselling. When I saw her again some time later she was in a good relationship and was thinking of getting married for the first time in her life. This was clear testimony that she had indeed healed.

SUMMARY

The digestive system is sometimes described as the weak point of the body. It is certainly a vulnerable point because it is intimately tied into our emotional state. However, when we unblock emotional energy because of suppressed anger or fear, it can become a power point in the body. Many healers refer to the solar plexus area as the source of our personal power and, having seen some amazing transformations in people, I can only agree with this.

The digestive tract is probably the most misunderstood part of our anatomy; it is extremely complex and very sensitive. It is the centre not just of our emotions and our immunity, but reflects the level of sensitivity of the person. By that I mean that the more highly sensitive one is, the more the digestive system will react to negative foods such as sugar, caffeine, stimulants, food additives.

Many people with digestive problems have an underlying emotional problem. In order to heal, you have to tackle not only the surface manifestation, i.e. the physical symptoms, but also the underlying emotions.

6

DIGESTIVE PROBLEMS CAN AFFECT OTHER PARTS OF THE BODY

You are aware by now that digestive disturbances can cause problems elsewhere in the body and are seldom limited to the digestive tract. We say that these effects are secondary to an underlying digestive disturbance. As you will learn in this chapter, these secondary effects can disturb almost any other system in the body — the muscular, skeletal, endocrine, nervous, respiratory, urinary, and genital systems as well as the skin. These secondary effects can be as varied as sleep disturbances in one person and arthritis in another. What is interesting is that many people present to their practitioner with the secondary effect, e.g. a skin rash or decreased sex drive, and are often unaware of the underlying digestive problem. This is because the digestive tract can be quite silent when in difficulty; it is poorly supplied with nerves when compared with the skin, for example, and so does not give strong warning signs when something is wrong. The skin by comparison will give you instant and strong messages when even something minor happens, e.g. a pin prick. There can be advanced disease such as cancer in the colon (large intestine) and the only symptom that the patient might be complaining of is a change in bowel habit i.e. constipation or diarrhoea. So, it is often these secondary effects of intestinal problems that bring people to see their doctor or health practitioner.

A malfunctioning digestive system underlies so many medical problems. This is because it has the potential to become very toxic from food left too long in the intestines or poorly digested by the intestines. In the same way that food will decay quite rapidly if left at room temperature, food will 'go off' even faster at body temperature. This is why all the health spas across the world focus on bowel cleansing and this is why all the health magazines speak about detoxification. The intestinal tract is the key to good health and to retarding the ageing process. This is why almost every culture on the planet has fasting as part of it; for example, I grew up in Ireland having to fast during Lent, the Muslims have Ramadan and so on. It is strange, however, that we pay so little attention to our diet and to the process of digestion and rather take it so much for granted.

Digestive Problems Can Affect the Liver

All nutrients that are absorbed across the intestinal wall pass into the bloodstream. This nutrient-rich blood then passes along the portal vein to the liver where it is either metabolised — chemically broken down further to release energy — or stored. In addition to sorting out nutrients, the liver has to render anything toxic harmless to the body. It has a number of ways of doing this but the end result is substances that are incapable of harming the body. You can imagine the level of toxicity when the small intestine starts to ferment or putrefy food — most of the food will end up being converted into toxic chemicals such as indican, putrescine and nervine, instead of into nutrients. This high level of toxicity puts a tremendous workload on the liver as it tries to detoxify these chemicals. However, the liver has a limited capacity to deal with toxins, and when it becomes overburdened and cannot cope, the toxins then bypass the liver and get into the main circulation, where they can wreak havoc in other parts of the body, including the liver itself. This is how a digestive problem such as fermentation can stress the liver

103

and ultimately impair its ability to such an extent that it becomes inflamed and unable to function effectively.

Figure 6.1 *NUTRIENTS BEING TRANSPORTED FROM THE SMALL INTESTINE TO THE LIVER*

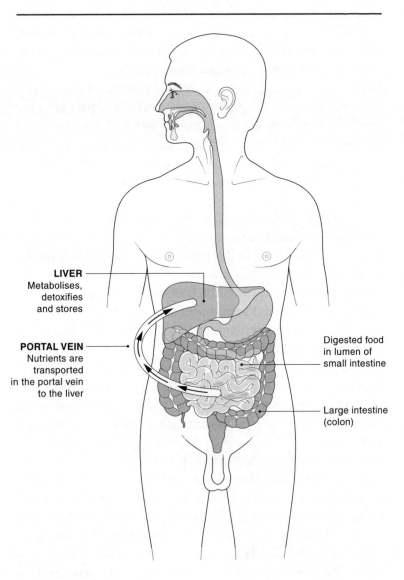

LIVER
Metabolises,
detoxifies
and stores

PORTAL VEIN
Nutrients are
transported
in the portal vein
to the liver

Digested food
in lumen of
small intestine

Large intestine
(colon)

The liver's main job is to release energy from food; when it becomes impaired one of the first symptoms is lack of energy. While not everyone with lack of energy necessarily has a liver problem — other causes include iron deficiency, low thyroid function, vitamin B_{12} deficiency, etc. — many people who suffer from fatigue who do not have any of these other conditions may well have a liver problem. The liver problem is most commonly secondary to an intestinal problem.

Figure 6.1 shows how all the nutrients in the lumen of the small intestine cross the intestinal wall and are then transported to the liver. In addition to these 'goodies', nasty toxic chemicals, the 'baddies', can also cross the intestinal wall and travel to the liver. If these chemicals are not detoxified they have the potential to disrupt many bodily functions.

DIGESTIVE PROBLEMS CAN AFFECT THE URINARY TRACT

When the liver is presented with toxic chemicals such as conventional drugs, poisons, chemical additives in food, or chemicals from decaying food in the intestine, it attempts to neutralise these chemicals. If the detoxifying function of the liver becomes overloaded, these toxins enter the general circulation. Having circulated around the body, the blood is then filtered by the kidneys and some of these toxins are removed and then pass out of the body in the urine. However, these chemicals can irritate the kidneys and bladder and cause urinary symptoms such as frequency of urination. Some of these chemicals irritate the bladder so much that the person has to pass water many times a day. These people will complain of a weak bladder or suggest that they have cystitis.

So, if you suffer from urinary frequency and there is no infection present, consider the possibility of toxicity. One helpful measure to use while treating the underlying cause of the toxicity is to dilute these toxins by drinking lots of water — two to three litres a day of purified water, as tap water can be quite toxic also.

In summary then, toxicity from the intestines can put strain on the liver and irritate the urinary tract (kidneys and bladder). Patients with high levels of toxicity often complain of low energy and urinary frequency.

DIGESTIVE PROBLEMS CAN AFFECT THE BRAIN

If you have a fermentation problem, the starchy foods that you eat will be converted to alcohols and aldehydes — chemicals that have a strong effect on the nervous system, especially the brain. (Remember that commercial alcohol such as wine and beer is made by fermenting a starch such as barley in the presence of yeast.)

In my book *Alternatives to Tranquillisers* I mentioned that the two most important micro-nutrients for the brain are B complex vitamins and magnesium. If these micro-nutrients are not absorbed from the intestine in sufficient quantities, the central nervous system will not function properly. Dysbiosis can result in a decrease in the supply of B vitamins available for absorption, and parasites such as *Giardia lamblia* rob you of a number of micro-nutrients including B vitamins, especially vitamin B_{12}.

So, digestive problems can impair brain function. Symptoms that may result include impaired memory and concentration, feeling spacey, depression, irritability.

Your mood is controlled by chemicals in the brain called neurotransmitters. Toxins from the gut can alter the levels of these neurotransmitters, thereby bringing about not just a change in mood but also in alertness, vision, short-term memory, and sensitivity to sound and touch (see Figure 6.2). People who are toxic can manifest these and may find it difficult to get an explanation for them. If you have any of these symptoms, seek help from a practitioner of natural medicine.

Figure 6.2 *TOXINS CAN DISRUPT BRAIN CHEMISTRY*

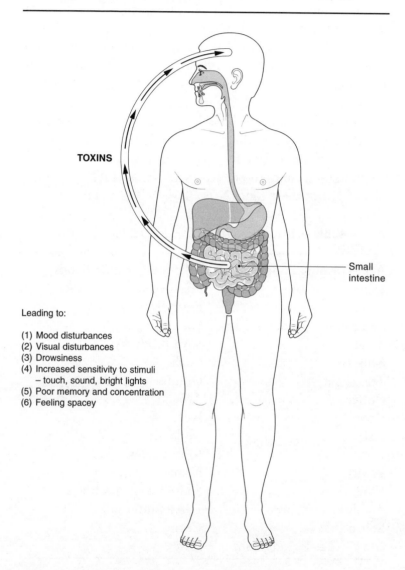

TOXINS

Small intestine

Leading to:

(1) Mood disturbances
(2) Visual disturbances
(3) Drowsiness
(4) Increased sensitivity to stimuli
 – touch, sound, bright lights
(5) Poor memory and concentration
(6) Feeling spacey

DIGESTIVE PROBLEMS CAN AFFECT THE SKIN

It is not uncommon today to see children with an acidic type of rash on the skin, especially on the face and arms. An acidic rash gives the skin a sandpaper feel, as small crystals are deposited on the skin and feel rough to the touch. Many children have such a rash because their bloodstream is acidic, usually as a result of diet or digestive problems. Many of these children have had antibiotics for ear infections, tonsillitis or chest infections, which can cause dysbiosis in the intestines. Dysbiosis causes cravings for sugary foods, bread, biscuits, etc., all of which are acidic foods. It is therefore very important to control the diet of such children, especially for the first few months, to allow the pH of the blood to return to normal. I prefer a diet consisting of 80 per cent alkaline foods and 20 per cent acid foods. Table 6.1 below gives a list of these foods.

Table 6.1 *ACID- AND ALKALINE-FORMING FOODS*

Acid-Forming Foods	Alkaline-Forming Foods
Sugar	Fresh vegetables (most)
Flour	Fresh fruits (most)
Flour-based products	Honey
Meat	Soya products
Milk	Garlic
Tea	Onions
Coffee	Avocados
Eggs	Nuts
Fish	Molasses
Pasta	Mushrooms
Poultry	Salads
Vinegar	Soured dairy products
Alcohol	(e.g buttermilk)
Soft drinks	Corn
Most drugs (e.g. aspirin)	Dates

Other common skin problems that I see are ringworm, athlete's foot and jock itch, all of which are manifestations of a fungal infection. GPs tend to treat the skin condition and leave it at that; practitioners of natural medicine treat the digestive tract and then the skin. This is because fungal infections are almost always a manifestation of intestinal dysbiosis. Therefore it is more important to treat the underlying dysbiosis than to treat the skin, because treating the dysbiosis alone will ultimately solve the skin problem. Hence, there is really no need to treat ringworm or athlete's foot topically, but, having said that, many practitioners will treat the itch associated with such rashes and some will use anti-fungal creams as well.

A good indicator of the presence of intestinal dysbiosis is a fungal infection of the toenails, which usually presents as discolouration of the nail. When examining someone I always check the feet for nail infections and for fungal infections between the toes. A fungal infection of the nail presents as a whitish coating on the surface of the nail, or as a greenish/yellowish discolouration or as thickening of the nail. Painting tea tree oil onto the nail can be very helpful for such infections, but again one has to check for intestinal dysbiosis.

DIGESTIVE PROBLEMS CAN AFFECT THE JOINTS

Most textbooks on natural medicine emphasise the role of diet and digestive problems in the development of arthritis. Indeed, conventional medical textbooks also note the link between arthritis and certain bowel problems such as ulcerative colitis. What is this link?

Toxins from the bowel can bypass an overworked or impaired liver and so enter the circulation. They are then often deposited in the muscles and joints, setting up an inflammatory response as the body tries to reject them. This inflammatory response causes the area to become red, hot and sore. Painkillers and anti-inflammatories can alleviate the symptoms but they do nothing to solve the underlying toxicity problem; indeed, because the drugs have to be detoxified by the liver they can add to the toxicity problem. In addition, these drugs can damage the lining of the intestinal tract, thereby aggravating the problem even further. Now you see why naturopaths and homeopaths scorn the use of such drugs. Again, as with the skin, it is important to treat the underlying intestinal problem, as well as alleviating the pain by using acupuncture or herbal painkillers, such as white willow or meadowsweet.

DIGESTIVE PROBLEMS CAN AFFECT THE HORMONAL SYSTEM

Hormonal disturbances and digestive problems are inter-linked. Digestive problems can upset the hormonal system and vice versa. Earlier in this book you learned that increased levels of the stress hormones, adrenaline and cortisone, can disturb intestinal function. Taking the contraceptive pill, which has two hormones — oestrogen and progesterone — can disturb the ecology of the small intestine and upset the bacterial population. Men suffering from intestinal dysbio-sis can experience a drop in their testosterone levels resulting in decreased sex drive; women suffering from dysbiosis also experience hormonal imbalances resulting in pre-menstrual tension and other menstrual irregularities.

Intestinal dysbiosis is also associated with sub-clinical hypothyroidism, in which the level of thyroid hormone (thy-roxine) is reduced but not sufficiently to show up on blood tests. Hypothyroidism slows the metabolism and so drops one's energy level.

As you can see, the digestive and hormonal systems are interlinked; in fact, the whole process of digestion is entirely under the control of the hormonal system. The release of digestive juices and enzymes is triggered by certain hormones, e.g. gastrin stimulates the release of gastric juices from the cells lining the stomach wall. These digestive hormones are in turn affected by the levels of other hor-mones in the bloodstream and in this way one has an effect on the other. Hence it is easy to understand how the two systems — digestive and hormonal — are so interlinked.

DIGESTIVE PROBLEMS CAN AFFECT OTHER PARTS OF THE BODY

Dysbiosis can cause oral thrush and vaginal thrush; it can also cause vaginitis, vaginal itching and vaginal discharge.

In men, inflammation of the prostate gland can be caused by systemic dysbiosis, as can decreased sexual libido. This latter problem can cause strain in a relationship, as the person's partner can misinterpret it as rejection.

Toxins from the intestines circulating in the bloodstream can deposit in the muscles, causing muscle aches and pains. As you will read shortly in one of the case histories, this can hinder one's ability to exercise. Some people with dysbiosis can also experience muscle twitching. I remember one patient whose lower eyelid used to twitch for up to thirty minutes at a time. It did not bother her but she could never find an explanation for it. It disappeared once she treated the dysbiosis.

Because every cell in the body needs goodies, i.e. nutrients and oxygen supplied by the bloodstream, every cell can potentially be damaged by toxins, the baddies, in the bloodstream. Hence, toxins from the digestive tract have the potential to impair almost any bodily function.

DIGESTIVE PROBLEMS CAN CAUSE VITAMIN/MINERAL DEFICIENCIES

The billions of good bacteria lining the intestinal tract produce a range of B vitamins. These can be absorbed across the intestinal wall into the bloodstream and supplement the B vitamin supply from our diet. If these good bacteria are replaced with bad bacteria and parasites, we not only lose the supply of B vitamins, but the bad bacteria and parasites rob us of essential micro-nutrients (e.g. zinc and vitamin B_{12}). For example, the common intestinal parasite *Giardia lamblia* depletes us of all the B vitamins, zinc and copper. The two organs most in need of zinc are the pancreas and the prostate gland — the two 'Ps' — and so a deficiency in zinc can predispose one to diabetes, prostatitis and enlargement of the prostate gland. Zinc is a very important antioxidant for every cell in the body; it is also a co-factor in many enzyme reactions in the liver.

Mouth ulcers are common in people with advanced dysbiosis, as they are caused by a vitamin deficiency, especially B vitamins. Hence, everyone who has intestinal dysbiosis should take a good multi-vitamin and multi-mineral supplement. If left untreated, intestinal problems can cause significant micro-nutrient deficiencies.

CASE HISTORY — JEAN: MOUTH ULCERS

Jean, a primary school teacher, had been suffering from mouth ulcers for years. In the past year in particular they were almost continuous and were very painful. She was at her wits' end, having tried many different approaches — multi-vitamins, pharmaceutical gels (containing an antibiotic and an analgesic), coating the lining of the mouth with live yoghurt, homeopathic and herbal remedies. Some of these measures helped in the short-term but did not effect a cure.

Having met a number of cases like Jean's in the past, I asked about antibiotic usage and if she had been on the pill prior to the onset of mouth ulcers. She told me that she had had a hysterectomy eight years ago and because of a post-operative infection she was given intravenous and later oral antibiotics for about three weeks. It was after this that the mouth ulcers began.

Her stool analysis revealed a 3+ overgrowth of two species of fungi, as well as the cysts of the parasite *Giardia lamblia*. The urine sample suggested gut fermentation. It was no wonder she could not find permanent improvement from the above measures, as she had a very significant digestive disturbance. I treated her intensively for the next three months using the gut fermentation diet and digestive aids, as well as anti-fungal treatment and a probiotic. At the end of this period of time her digestive tract had improved and she herself felt a lot better; the mouth ulcers had cleared away and did not return. I then suggested that she continue with the probiotic and multi-vitamin/multi-mineral supplement and broaden her diet but to stay away from all refined carbohydrates. To date she has remained ulcer-free.

If you have had one or more courses of antibiotics it is important that you have a stool analysis done, especially if you have any of the symptoms mentioned in this book. Jean would never have got to the bottom of her problem if this test had not been done. Remember that fermentation and dysbiosis can take time to treat and a lot of commitment, so be patient. As in Jean's case the rewards can be tremendous.

CASE HISTORY — PATRICK: MUSCLE WEAKNESS

Patrick was a successful accountant and loved running in his spare time. He was very competitive and used to run half and sometimes full marathons. Every evening he used to train on the roads and in the gym, but of late he felt that his muscles were getting weaker and on occasion were quite painful as well. He also tired more quickly and felt that he just did not have the stamina any longer. This did not make sense to him as he was only thirty-two years old and was in excellent health. The only relevant piece of history was the chronic stress that he was under in trying to build a successful company.

His tests showed that he was suffering from gut fermentation, although he had little in the way of abdominal symptoms. I treated him by using the gut fermentation diet plus nutritional and homeopathic supplements, warning him that because of the low carbohydrate intake during the first month of treatment he would have to cut down on the amount of exercise. I saw him monthly thereafter and his progress was excellent. It took three months in all before he could compete again in marathons but the improvement in muscle weakness and pain was felt within days of commencing treatment.

Muscle weakness is not necessarily symptomatic of a muscle problem; it is more commonly due to toxins being deposited in the muscles. These toxins interfere with the functioning of the muscle cells, causing weakness, cramps, pain and twitching.

This is an excellent example of how intestinal problems can be silent and how it is often the secondary effect, in this case muscle weakness, that the patient presents with. Because muscles have such a rich blood supply, they are often the site where toxins are deposited. Anyone who treats neck and back problems — masseurs, aromatherapists, physiotherapists — will be all too aware of this. If you have a neck or back problem or suffer from muscle problems elsewhere, have your doctor do the appropriate tests to rule out an intestinal problem.

CASE HISTORY — AHMED: PROSTATITIS

Ahmed was forty years old and had persistent prostatitis which was not responding to conventional treatment — mainly antibiotics. He then decided to read up on it and to treat himself with natural medicines. When I met him he was on many supplements, including saw palmetto, pygeum africanum, amino acids, zinc and antioxidants. He came to me because he was worried that there was something else going on, as nothing seemed to help.

After examining him and doing extensive tests it was clear that this was not a prostate problem, as the prostate was completely normal on examination and the tests confirmed this. The stool test and blood test revealed severe dysbiosis. I could not state categorically that this was the cause of the prostate symptoms, but we agreed to observe any changes in his symptoms while treating the dysbiosis. His improvement was slow, as he found the diet very difficult to stick to and it took him almost a month to get his head around it, so to speak. Once he had mentally adjusted to the diet he showed steady improvement. After three months of treatment his symptoms were gone completely for the first time in twelve months. He felt very grateful to me as I had saved him so much expense in herbal and nutritional supplements and in avoiding the costly medical tests that his GP had suggested.

Ahmed's case was very straightforward and again illustrates the connection between the digestive tract and seemingly unconnected symptoms elsewhere in the body.

CASE HISTORY — JACKIE: SKIN ITCHING

Jackie was twenty-one years old and her only complaint was episodes of intense skin itching, which had begun nine months previously. This itching, which had no accompanying rash, affected any part of her skin but most commonly the arms and legs. She was otherwise in good health. The only important piece of history was that she had been on the pill for two years continuously. Since the pill can cause dysbiosis I checked for it and sure enough she had a mild case of it. I treated the dysbiosis and within two weeks of commencing treatment the itch was gone and to date has not returned. As Jackie continued to avoid sugary foods and take a probiotic, it is not unreasonable then to suggest that the itching was caused by intestinal dysbiosis.

I am not suggesting that all cases of prostatitis, skin itching or muscle weakness are caused by digestive disturbances. What I am trying to point out is that digestive problems can cause secondary symptoms in other parts of the body. Therefore, it is prudent to always check for an intestinal problem almost regardless of the symptoms you may have. The digestive tract is *the* major source of toxicity in the body and has the potential to create symptoms in any other system of the body.

OTHER IMPORTANT SYMPTOMS

The above case histories illustrate a few secondary symptoms associated with digestive problems. However, there are others that I have not mentioned; I have listed these below in Table 6.2. If you are experiencing any of these symptoms get checked out by your local practitioner.

Table 6.2 *SECONDARY SYMPTOMS OF A DIGESTIVE PROBLEM*

Fatigue	Bad breath
Mood swings	Glossitis
Poor memory and concentration	Urinary frequency
Skin rashes	Joint pain
Body odour	Vaginal discharge

SUMMARY

Some of the symptoms associated with a digestive disturbance are experienced in other parts of the body; these are called secondary symptoms. The association with the digestive tract is often missed by the doctor or practitioner and instead the symptom is treated in isolation. This results in recurrences of the symptoms and frustrates both patient and practitioner.

Because the intestinal tract has such a profound effect on all other parts of the body, it is essential to rule out a digestive disturbance in anyone complaining of the symptoms that I have outlined in this chapter. Insist on having the proper tests done, including a stool and urine test, especially if you have been on the pill, antibiotics, steroids or anti-inflammatory drugs.

7

TREATMENT OF COMMON DIGESTIVE COMPLAINTS

This chapter will deal with the treatment of some common digestive complaints using natural medicine. You will see that diet plays a very big role, irrespective of the complaint. The purpose of using a diet is not to lose weight or to make your life more difficult or to punish you for bad eating habits, etc; the sole purpose is to reduce the level of toxicity in your body. This is achieved by removing potentially harmful foods from the diet, e.g. refined carbohydrates (especially sugar), food additives (some of which are carcinogenic), and stimulants such as tea, coffee and caffeine (these disturb the involuntary nervous system — coffee also strips away the lining of mucus that protects the cells of the digestive tract). Toxicity is reduced by shifting the acid/alkaline balance in the body towards a more neutral or alkaline pH. Too many people on a Western diet are very acidic, as they consume too many acid-forming foods and too few alkaline foods. You can refer to a list of these foods on page 108 of this book. One common feature in following any diet is that somewhere along the line you will break it. This is an important part of the learning process, because reverting to the old diet can cause a severe reaction and it is by experiencing this reaction that you learn the importance of being on a diet. Many people beat themselves up for having broken a diet; rather learn from it, see it as a positive thing and then try again with greater understanding and commitment.

Diet is a common thread in treating digestive complaints, but using probiotics is another. Why do we need to use probiotics? If you consider that 90 per cent of the cells in your body are actually bacteria and not human cells you might well be shocked. Ninety percent of you is not you at all. Put another way, only 10 per cent of your body cells are actually human cells. So to say that the bacterial population that lines the tubes of the body as well as the surface of the body is important is a bit of an understatement; it is critical. When this bacterial population is disturbed it can lead to many digestive complaints; indeed, it can lead to many wide-ranging medical conditions, as you learned in the last chapter. Therefore, one of the priorities in treatment is to restore this bacterial population back to normal. That is why we use probiotics, as they contain lots of 'good' bacteria.

We are supposed to use them every day to maintain good health. Probiotics are used by people the world over in some form — e.g. when I was growing up we used buttermilk, the Fulani in West Africa use curded milk, the black population of southern Africa use soured milk, and so on. The older doctors used to advocate the use of live yoghurt, but the younger modern doctors have not been taught its importance and do not educate patients to use it.

One substance that I will speak about quite a lot in this chapter is an amino acid called glutamine. Glutamine is the main nutrient for the cells that line the digestive tract and so it is a very important addition to any treatment regimen. By boosting the nutrition of this delicate lining, you are allowing the digestive tract to heal. Glutamine is also the precursor of an important chemical in all cells of the body; this chemical is called glutathione and it protects the cells from damage by toxins and viruses. So feeding the cells lots of glutamine helps protect them from damage.

With severe or advanced disease it is important to use

foods that are easy to digest and absorb, thereby reducing the workload of the digestive tract. This also applies to vitamin and mineral supplements, which are easier to absorb if taken as food (e.g. spirulina and alfalfa are rich in vitamins and minerals) rather than as tablets. It is also very important to go slowly and allow lots of time for healing to occur, as the digestive tract is a very long structure — 30 feet approximately. With advanced disease it is also important not to aggravate the condition, so using bland, soft foods makes sense initially, as well as weaker strengths of medicines. Also use weaker strengths of probiotics and prebiotics such as fructo-oligosaccharide (FOS). Altering the bacterial population too quickly can cause lots of bloating and wind and may cause diarrhoea. If you experience any aggravations during treatment, just halve the dosage of the medicines you are taking as this will often alleviate the problem; if this does not work then seek help.

Another useful piece of advice is to very slowly reduce any conventional medicines that you may have been on prior to treatment with natural medicines; in other words, do not stop them suddenly but rather give the body a chance to adjust by reducing them slowly.

Above I mentioned that many people are too acidic, i.e. the pH of their blood and saliva is too low. To help shift this pH balance I advocate the use of alkaline salts — sodium bicarbonate, potassium bicarbonate, etc. I also advocate drinking lots of water as well as lemon juice and honey to alkalinise the system; in some people I recommend the use of apple cider vinegar for the same reason. If you wish to check the pH of your saliva, just go to your local pharmacy and ask for litmus paper. Saliva pH should be between 6.2 and 6.4. If your reading is less than 6.0 you are too acidic and in need of treatment.

Let's now look at how to treat some of the more common conditions affecting the digestive system. I shall begin at the mouth and work downwards.

Mouth Ulcers (Aphthous Ulcers)

These are quite common and most of us will have experienced them at some stage of our lives. However, for some people they can be a real problem as they recur and can be very painful.

Mouth ulcers are commonly associated with intestinal dysbiosis. However, not everyone with mouth ulcers has dysbiosis. Other causes include nutritional deficiencies — vitamin B deficiency as well as iron and zinc deficiency — food allergies, especially to gluten, and stress.

Treatment involves correcting the cause, i.e. treating the dysbiosis or correcting any nutritional deficiency and eliminating any foods that you are allergic to. Stress management is an essential therapy for anyone under ongoing stress. When correcting an iron deficiency it is important to use a non-constipating form of iron, since many of the conventional iron tablets cause constipation. Good non-constipating forms of iron include Floradix Herbal Iron Supplement and Solgar's Gentle Iron.

Bad Breath (Halitosis)

Bad breath is more commonly associated with digestive problems such as fermentation and dysbiosis than with any other type of problem. It is less commonly associated with dental problems such as tooth infections, periodontal disease or poor dental hygiene.

Treatment involves checking for a digestive disturbance and treating it effectively. Chronic constipation can be treated with natural medicines such as linseed oil, senna and in severe cases, cascara. Stomach acid levels should be checked and, if these are low, treated with betaine hydrochloride, which should be used with each meal. If no evidence of a digestive disturbance is found, then go to a dentist who can check for amalgam leakage from fillings and other causes of halitosis.

PEPTIC ULCER

Most of you will be aware that it is now believed that peptic ulcers are caused by a particular bacterium called *Helicobacter pylori* and not by excess stomach acid as was once thought. Conventional medical treatment involves the use of antibiotics to kill this bacterium. It is very strange to find bacteria growing in an extremely acid environment, so it is more likely that people with a peptic ulcer have low stomach acid — remember that both high and low stomach acid levels give exactly the same symptoms, so they are hard to distinguish. Most people with peptic ulcers have been under stress, and since stress lowers the secretion of stomach acid it is more likely that anyone with a peptic ulcer has low stomach acid; strangely, however, this is not always the case.

The bacterium *Helicobacter* is found in 80 per cent of people with duodenal and gastric ulcers and with gastritis. In the general population this bacterium is found in 30 per cent of people but only 10 per cent will experience symptoms. This raises a number of important questions, e.g. if this bacterium were the only cause of stomach ulcers, then everyone with a peptic ulcer would have it — so what about the 20 per cent who have ulcers but not the bacterium? And why do some people who have the bacterium go on to develop ulcers and others do not? It would seem that the cause of digestive ulcers is multi-factorial and not just merely the consequences of a bacterial infection.

Some of you may be aware of the work of Dr Batmanghelidj, who was able to treat peptic ulcers with water alone while he was in prison in Iran. His work has now become well known around the world. He suggests that for the cells of the stomach to produce sufficient mucus to protect themselves from the acid environment in the stomach, they need lots of water. This makes a lot of sense. Since 70 per cent of the human body is water, each cell of the body needs water if it is to function efficiently. So drink lots of water daily.

There are excellent natural medicines to help anyone suffering from either gastritis or a peptic ulcer. Firstly, however, let us take a look at diet and lifestyle measures that will help.

DIET

This is the most important mode of treatment, because none of the other therapies will work unless one's diet is altered. General measures include the following:

a) drink six to eight glass of water daily
b) take small meals frequently
c) chew the food very well
d) alkalinise the system with alkaline salts
e) eat foods that are easy to digest — soups, fish, steamed or stir-fried or baked vegetables, baby food
f) eliminate the worst acid-forming foods — gluten, cheese, sugar, tomatoes
g) eliminate coffee, as it strips the mucus lining from the digestive tract
h) eliminate all spicy foods, cigarettes and alcohol
i) do not use drugs that damage the lining of the digestive tract, such as aspirin, and all the anti-inflammatory drugs — brufen, voltaren, ponstan, etc.
j) exercise once a day but do a form of exercise that you enjoy.

NUTRITIONAL SUPPLEMENTS

L-glutamine. This is one of the most popular anti-ulcer medications available today. It has been clinically proven to assist the healing of peptic ulcers, gastritis, irritable bowel syndrome and colitis. It is the main nutrient for cells lining the digestive tract and it helps parts of this tract that have been damaged to heal. Use two grams three times daily between meals.

HERBAL MEDICINES

Liquorice root. This is the most important herbal medicine used to heal ulcers. It has shown impressive clinical results in the treatment of gastric and duodenal ulcers; in fact, its effectiveness was found to be superior to anti-ulcer drugs. Liquorice stimulates mucus production, which protects the cells from damage; it also enhances blood flow, thereby speeding up the healing process.

It is best to use deglycyrrhised liquorice (this is ordinary liquorice root that has had the chemical glycyrrhic acid removed), as glycyrrhic acid has the effect of raising the blood pressure. Since some people have undiagnosed high blood pressure it is safer to use the deglycyrrhised form, which is often abbreviated to DGL. In terms of dosage use 500–1500 mg of standardised extract thirty minutes before meals.

Grapefruit seed extract. This is an extract made from the seeds and the pulp of grapefruit. Like grapefruit, it has quite a bitter taste. It has proven anti-bacterial properties and so will suppress the growth of *Helicobacter pylori.* Use 15 drops in a glass of water three times daily.

Psyllium husks. The combination of soluble and insoluble fibre in psyllium seed husks reduces the transit time for food to pass through the intestinal tract as well as helping to bind toxins that might otherwise accelerate damage to the lining of the digestive tract. In people with duodenal ulcers a high-fibre diet has been shown to reduce the risk of recurrence. Take two grams twice daily between meals.

HOMEOPATHY

I have focused on four remedies below and I shall describe the type of person most suited to each remedy.

Pulsatilla. This remedy works best in shy, gentle people who are prone to changeable moods, who are fair-haired and who prefer cool weather and fresh air. Use a 6c potency frequently if the symptoms are acute, e.g. every 15 minutes; otherwise use three times daily. Use one tablet or 10 drops as the standard dosage. This dosage is the same for the following three remedies.

Sepia. This remedy works best in people who are easily depressed and worn out and who are dark-haired and have sallow skin. Sepia is a remedy most often used in females but not exclusively.

Argentum nitricum. This remedy works best in thin people who are anxious and who comfort eat, especially on refined carbohydrates.

Graphite. This is suited to overweight people who have coarse features and whose skin is dry and rough. They tend to prefer outdoor jobs and often have skin problems such as eczema or psoriasis.

GALL-STONES

The main cause of gall-stones is too much animal fat — butter, cheese, bacon, meat, eggs — in the diet. Many people have small gall-stones in the gall-bladder but they do not cause problems. Others have gall-stones that cause major problems. For example, a stone can get stuck in the neck of the gall-bladder, completely obstructing the flow of bile. In an attempt to overcome this blockage the gall-bladder contracts very vigorously, causing intense pain. The pain is located under the right rib-cage and radiates into the back or to the tip of the right shoulder. Vomiting often accompanies the pain.

Smaller blockages in the neck of the gall-bladder or in the duct leading from the gall-bladder down to the small intestine may cause similar but less intense symptoms; jaundice may also occur.

Diagnosis is made with the help of ultrasound, which will outline clearly any stones present. In conventional medicine removal of the gall-bladder is the main form of treatment. However, stones may also be shattered by lithotripsy which uses sound waves to break up the stones.

DIET

In natural medicine the best form of treatment involves taking 3 tablespoons of olive oil with the juice of one lemon last thing at night and first thing upon rising the next morning. This treatment will flush out the stones. Thereafter it is wise to avoid all animal fats and use only cold-pressed vegetable oils, e.g. virgin olive oil, linseed oil, etc. Drink lots of pure water — six to eight glasses daily.

HERBAL MEDICINE

Berberis vulgaris (barberry). This is an excellent herb to ease the flow of bile and to ease liver congestion. Use 3 ml of pure tincture three times daily in a little water.

Chelidonium. This is another excellent remedy to assist where there are stones in the gall-bladder or inflammation anywhere in the biliary tract. Use 3 ml of pure tincture three times daily in a little water.

ACUPUNCTURE

This is particularly useful for relieving the pain associated with an acute attack. Use the following acupressure or acupuncture points: Gall-bladder 26, 34 and 40, as well as Liver 7 and 13.

IRRITABLE BOWEL SYNDROME (IBS)

This is quite a common intestinal disorder affecting over 10 per cent of the population. It is also called spastic colon, mucous colitis and functional bowel disorder. The main symptoms are abdominal pain, bloating and abnormal bowel movements, i.e. diarrhoea alternating with constipation. No cause has been found.

DIET

This is of critical importance and must precede any other form of treatment by at least four to six weeks. The aim of the diet is to reduce toxicity and to eliminate foods that the patient might be allergic to. The aim is also to be as gentle as possible, as an inflamed digestive tract is very sensitive to any aggravation, including some natural medicines. This is why I recommend leaving a gap of four to six weeks before commencing on any medicines.

For the first month use Stage 1 of the gut fermentation diet and use a digestive enzyme with each meal to improve digestion. In the second month, continue with Stage 1 of the diet and introduce L-glutamine, 1–2 grams three times daily between meals. I also add in a mild probiotic as well as either linseed oil capsules or the oil itself, as the capsules can be an irritant. In the third month, broaden the diet but still exclude all gluten, all yeast and all sugars. Continue with the above medications but increase the glutamine to two grams three times daily and use a stronger probiotic. If any food item or medication causes an aggravation I tend to wait a little longer before re-introducing it. Try sourdough bread but chew it very well. If the bread is well tolerated continue with it. I continue with such a diet and medicines for a minimum of six months and longer if necessary.

NUTRITIONAL SUPPLEMENTS

Calcium and Magnesium. These two salts have definite antispasmodic properties and have been used to prevent and alleviate muscle spasms associated with IBS. Use a supplement that has approximately twice as much calcium as magnesium, e.g. 1000 mg of calcium and 500 mg of magnesium.

L-Glutamine. This is an amino acid that has the power to heal the digestive lining and so should be used in large quantities for the duration of treatment. I would recommend a dosage of approximately two grams three times daily between meals; it may be wiser to start at half this dosage for the first few weeks and then increase it. It is a very safe substance and some people use up to 20 g daily.

Probiotics. Gradually increase the strength with time. Start with acidophilus alone and then add in bifidus later. Remember that it takes months for the bacterial flora to normalise, so persist. Keep all probiotic supplements in the fridge.

Prebiotics. These are substances that encourage the growth of 'good' bacteria. One example of a prebiotic is the sugar fructo-oligosaccharide (FOS). It can be very helpful, but start with a very low dosage, say one-quarter of a teaspoon daily, gradually building up to one teaspoon twice daily. The problem with FOS is it can cause a lot of wind and therefore discomfort in the bowel, so go slowly.

Digestive enzymes. If these are not produced in sufficient quantities, it can lead to food allergies, incomplete digestion and fermentation and putrefaction as well as dysbiosis, all of which may play a role in IBS. It is therefore important to take digestive enzymes with each meal — this may reduce the symptoms of IBS significantly. Follow the instructions on the leaflet; generally use one or two capsules depending on the size of the meal.

COLONIC IRRIGATION

This is also called colon hydrotherapy and it is extremely helpful for a number of digestive problems; it is particularly helpful for people suffering from IBS. I often refer patients with IBS for colonic irrigation whilst following the above regimen of treatment. It helps to detoxify the system quickly. Many patients feel an immediate benefit after it is performed. I discuss this therapy in detail on pages 141–2 of this book.

STRESS-RELIEVING TECHNIQUES

Learning to control anxiety is difficult but of enormous benefit. Exercise, breathing, self-hypnosis and biofeedback are quite simple techniques that can have significant impact.

If these techniques prove not to be sufficiently helpful, it is important then to seek help from a counsellor or psychologist.

DIVERTICULAR DISEASE

Diverticulae are small pouches that develop in the wall of the colon or large intestine. In the Western world 40 per cent of people over the age of sixty have them. Over 80 per cent of these people with diverticulae have no symptoms whatsoever. The most common complication of diverticular disease is infection and it is at this point that we use the term 'diverticulitis'. Infection occurs when a small piece of stool gets stuck in one of the pouches — see Figure 7.1 below. Diverticulitis is almost always associated with chronic constipation.

Figure 7.1 *DIVERTICULITIS*

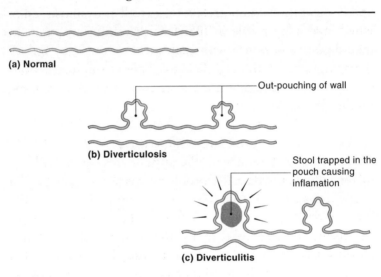

(a) Normal

Out-pouching of wall

(b) Diverticulosis

Stool trapped in the pouch causing inflamation

(c) Diverticulitis

DIET

Treatment is pretty much the same as for constipation. i.e. high-fibre diet, exercise, psyllium, linseed oil. It is also a good idea to use glutamine to heal the lining of the colon and also to use a probiotic.

HOMEOPATHY

There are a number of homeopathic remedies that are used, depending on the symptoms. Here are some of the remedies used.

Belladonna. A good remedy for people who get sudden gripping pain, especially on the left side of the abdomen.

Bryonia. Appropriate for people who experience a sharp stitch on the left side of the abdomen and who feel as if the abdomen is going to burst.

Colocynthis. Used for people who experience cramps, which are eased by lying down with the knees drawn up to the chest. These people may also experience abdominal pain associated with diarrhoea.

CONSTIPATION

As a general rule, you should have a bowel motion after each meal, i.e. three times daily if you eat three meals a day. Most people have at least one motion a day but some can go for days without having any motion at all. If you do not have at least one motion a day you are suffering from constipation.

Some doctors define constipation as the passage of a hard stool. Rather, it is the frequency with which you go to the toilet that is all-important, as you will learn below.

When you eat food it passes from the mouth down the oesophagus and into the stomach. The stomach then tells the colon to empty. This communication between the top end of the digestive tract and the bottom end is called the 'gastro-colic reflex' (see Figure 7.2). In other words, the top end tells the bottom end that it must empty as there is food entering the top end. This gastro-colic reflex works well in people who eats lots of roughage, such as wholegrain breads, muesli, wholegrain rice, lots of fruit and vegetables, etc. I lived for many years in different parts of Africa where people eat a very natural diet full of very fibrous foods — yams, cassava, millet, corn, sorghum and other cereals. Some African people use the same cereal for all their meals, e.g. maize porridge for breakfast, cooked maize meal with vegetables for lunch and the same in the evening. The gastro-colic reflex works well in such people. However, people in the urban areas of Africa and in the West eat less fibrous, more refined foods and so suffer from chronic constipation.

Figure 7.2 *GASTRO-COLIC REFLEX*

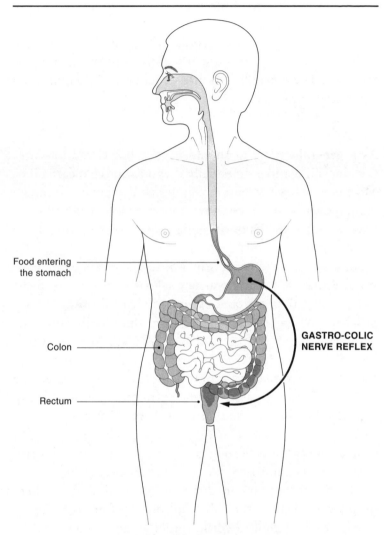

Food entering the stomach

Colon

Rectum

GASTRO-COLIC NERVE REFLEX

Top end (stomach) telling the bottom end (rectum) to empty

It is critically important to eliminate waste matter from the body. Food that is left to decay in your digestive system will produce nasty chemicals that can be poisonous to the body.

Hence, the single most important question to ask someone when assessing their level of health is the frequency with which they pass a bowel motion. This is why constipation is better defined as the failure to pass a bowel motion at least once a day.

Another reason why constipation is more common in the West is because we do not get enough physical activity. We spend long periods of time sitting in an office and then watching television in the evening. In contrast, people in the rural areas of Africa must walk long distances to get food, water, medical help, etc. They spend very little time sitting. Physical activity stimulates the bowel to function well and so assists elimination. So, if you eat a Western diet, add much more fibre to it and exercise at least every other day. About 90 per cent of cases of constipation can be helped purely by this simple adjustment in lifestyle.

Less common causes of constipation include anxiety, pregnancy, drugs (iron tablets, painkillers, and antidepressants), piles and anal fissures, low thyroid function. A change in bowel habit may be the first sign of colon cancer. Anyone over the age of fifty with a recent complaint of constipation (or diarrhoea) should be referred for medical tests to rule out cancer.

DIET

Introduce more wholegrains, vegetables (raw or slightly stir-fried) and fruit to the diet. Prunes and apricots have laxative properties so add these to the diet also.

EXERCISE

Vigorous exercise on alternate days, or better still daily, will help not just constipation but will give your whole body a wonderful boost.

WATER

Most people do not drink enough water and yet water is the single most important nutrient that we consume. Try to get a water purifier, as tap water is too toxic in most parts of Europe. Water purifiers use a process called *reverse osmosis with de-ionisation*; this is really a mechanical duplication of how plants purify water. It eliminates all chemicals, pesticides, herbicides, drug residues, metals and bacteria. The company Pure H_2O produces a range of such purification systems. The reverse osmosis process is a filtering process and is widely used in dialysis units, which need highly purified water. Reverse osmosis alone does not kill microbes such as harmful bacteria, and the more modern dialysis units now combine reverse osmosis with de-ionisation. Drink a minumum of six to eight glasses of pure water daily if you wish to be healthy.

HERBAL SUPPLEMENTS

Linseed. This is one supplement that I commonly prescribe for my patients. It is the seed of the plant known as common flax. The seed contains mucilage which, when added to water, swells up, increasing in volume considerably. This 'bulking' action stimulates peristalsis in the bowel and so stimulates the rectum to empty. It was used by the ancient Greeks to treat constipation. The seeds are available in some supermarkets and all good healthfood shops. Use one or two tablespoons daily. Chew them or add them to breakfast cereal. Alternatively, use one or two linseed oil capsules daily.

Rhubarb. This is a wonderful herb to assist the colon to eliminate waste material. It can be taken as a herbal tincture or as dried powder, or just add rhubarb to your diet. Rhubarb contains *anthraquinones,* which irritate the gut lining causing it to move faeces along more quickly. If used as a tincture, use two millilitres three times daily.

INFLAMMATORY BOWEL DISEASE (IBD)
This is a term to describe Crohn's disease and ulcerative colitis. The hallmark of this condition is inflammation; when it affects only the colon it is called ulcerative colitis; when it

affects the whole of the digestive tract it is called Crohn's disease. Symptoms include abdominal pain, cramps and diarrhoea. These cardinal symptoms may be accompanied by fever, rectal bleeding, recurrent abscesses and loss of weight. Many people have mild symptoms, while others require hospitalisation, especially if the diarrhoea is severe and the patient becomes dehydrated. Symptoms can occur in bouts and can then be followed by periods of remission. The risk of colon cancer is higher in people with ulcerative colitis.

Inflammatory bowel disease is a condition affecting Westerners for the most part. I have yet to see IBD in an African person. Research has shown a correlation with smoking cigarettes and with eating lots of refined carbohydrates and fast foods.

DIET

Diet is the single most important form of treatment in IBD. Studies have shown a reduction in symptoms in people who adhere to a hypoallergenic diet — excluding foods that commonly cause allergies such as wheat, milk, soya, etc. Alternative medicine often approaches IBD as sensitisation dysbiosis, where food allergies have led to the onset of an auto-immune pathology, since IBD is an auto-immune disease. It is therefore very important to find out which foods are aggravating the patient's digestive system and then exclude those foods. However, there is no single diet that will work for everyone.

Having said that, studies on Crohn's disease in particular have shown that a low-sulphur diet works for many patients. This diet involves eliminating the following foods: eggs, cheese, milk, ice-cream, mayonnaise, soya, drinks with sulphur (e.g. wine), nuts, cruciferous vegetables (broccoli, cabbage, cauliflower, brussels sprouts). The research shows that a high percentage of the people who stuck to this diet did not suffer relapses.

HERBAL SUPPLEMENTS

Grapefruit seed extract, which has anti-microbial properties, is an excellent remedy in IBD. Many of the flare-ups in IBD are caused by infection with bacteria or parasites.

NUTRITIONAL SUPPLEMENTS

Glutamine is the single most important supplement to take. It helps the cells lining the digestive tract to heal. Use 2–4 grams three times daily.

Linseed oil is an omega three oil and so has anti-inflammatory properties. Use one or two tablespoons daily with food or use one or two capsules daily.

Probiotics are also important, as IBD is commonly associated with dysbiosis and is indeed regarded as a form of dysbiosis. Hence the treatment is the same as the treatment for dysbiosis (see Chapter 3).

HOMEOPATHY

I like to use homeopathics in this condition to minimise any aggravation, especially bleeding.

Phosphorus is useful, especially if there is pain or bleeding.

Mercurius corrosivus is helpful if the stool has an offensive odour and causes pain on defecating. It is also useful where there is diarrhoea and bleeding and great straining to pass small amounts of blood or mucus.

Arsenicum album is appropriate for people who are anxious and restless and who experience burning pain in the abdomen with vomiting, especially at night.

COLON CANCER

This is a common form of cancer in the Western world. The three main causes are: a) diet, b) dysbiosis and c) stress, but genetics seems to play a role in 5 to 10 per cent of people with this form of cancer.

Colon cancer is usually the end result of years of malfunctioning of the digestive tract. People who have suffered from long-standing constipation are more likely to develop cancer; also people who have had chronic dysbiosis are at increased risk. Most cancers are preceded by a period of great stress, e.g. the death of a loved one, divorce, etc. Cancer is also more common in people who are anxious and who suppress their emotions rather than express them.

Colon cancer is quite difficult to detect and so symptoms that are suggestive of it, such as loss of weight, change in bowel habit, blood in the stool, should be taken seriously. Because it is so difficult to detect, inspection of the colon by colonoscopy once a year for everyone over the age of fifty is good preventative medicine; this is obligatory for anyone with symptoms suggestive of colon cancer. Colonoscopy is the only way of diagnosing cancer of the colon.

The treatment of colon cancer really warrants a separate book but I shall briefly outline the principles of treatment.

DIET

The foods that constitute the greatest risk factors are saturated fats, meat (especially if it is grilled, barbecued or burned) and refined carbohydrates. Other risk factors include a diet low in fibre and low in vegetables, especially cruciferous vegetables (brussel sprouts, cabbage, cauliflower and broccoli). All cancer clinics around the world advocate eliminating all meat, particularly pork products, all refined carbohydrates, all fast foods, all sugar and all fats and oils, except for cold-pressed oils; these diets also advocate increasing the intake of vegetables, fruit, and soluble and insoluble fibre. There are many variations on this same dietary theme, such as the Moerman diet, which is very popular in Holland, and the Gerson diet, which is popular in the US and indeed in many other countries now.

COLONIC IRRIGATION/ENEMAS

Most cancer clinics around the world advocate the use of daily enemas to keep the bowel clear of faeces, thereby allowing the area to heal.

Some practitioners use enemas of butyrate — the salt of butyric acid — which actually makes a lot of common sense because butyric acid is the main nutrient utilised by the cells lining the colon. Others use coffee enemas, as coffee stimulates peristalsis and so assists bowel clearance.

Colonic irrigation is very helpful; not only does it clear the bowel out but probiotics or medicines such as tea tree oil can be inserted into the colon so ensuring that the good bacteria get to where they are required and any medicine can be placed where it is most needed.

The treatment that I outlined in Chapter 3 for dysbiosis is applicable to all patients with colon cancer.

NUTRITIONAL SUPPLEMENTS

Probiotics. Probiotics change dietary fibre into short-chain fatty acids, the most important of which is butyric acid. The short-chain fatty acids also have the effect of lowering the pH of the colon, thereby killing harmful bacteria. Probiotics also produce vitamin A, many B vitamins, and vitamin K; they also enhance peristalsis. They provide millions of good bacteria and are particularly important in people with cancer, as many of these people have an abnormal flora.

Antioxidants. All the antioxidant nutrients in high potency are very relevant in addition to calcium. Grape seed extract is the most powerful antioxidant, being fifty times more potent than vitamin C and twenty times more potent than vitamin E. Garlic oil capsules or raw garlic, mainly because of its anti-microbial effects, are very helpful too. Garlic and onions contain a nutrient called germanium which is believed to be the active ingredient in the healing waters of Lourdes.

Linseed oil is also helpful because of its bulking action on the stool.

HERBAL SUPPLEMENTS

Many herbs have anti-cancer properties. Probably the best known of these is mistletoe (*Viscum album*), but there are many others. One of the most famous herbal remedies is the Hoxsey tonic. This tonic contains a number of herbs in liquid and tablet form. Here is a list of the herbs in this formula:

Liquorice	Poke root
Red Clover	*Cascara amarga*
Burdock root	Prickly Ash bark
Stillingia root	Buckthorn bark
Berberis root	

This formula has been analysed by the National Cancer Institute and has been shown to have anti-cancer properties. In truth, it is always better to use herbs that are appropriate for the individual, rather than using prepared tonics; having said that, though, tonics can be enormously helpful.

OTHER THERAPIES

VISUALISATION

There are a number of books written about the power of visualisation, the most notable of which is *Getting Well Again* by Carl Simonton and his wife Stephanie. From their experience with hundreds of patients at their world-famous Cancer Counselling and Research Center in Dallas, Texas, the Simontons have demonstrated time and again the power of relaxation and visualisation to overcome cancer. They have described in their book how positive visual images and increased self-awareness can contribute to survival in cancer patients. Dr Simonton first used the visualisation technique in 1971 with a patient who had incurable cancer. Three times a day the patient practised a visualisation technique, which involved visualising his cancer as a group of weak, confused cells, growing out of control, and his white blood cells as highly organised soldiers attacking and destroying the cancer cells. He visualised his body removing the dead cells, his energy increasing and a feeling of well-being returning. This incurable patient overcame his cancer and is still alive today.

Since the Simontons' pioneering work in the 1970s, visualisation and guided imagery have become much more popular and accepted healing tools. There are many fine books to read on this topic but my favourite is *Creative Visualisation* by Shakti Gawain. If you haven't read this book or practised the wonderful exercises in visualisation that she mentions, I would urge you to do so as soon as possible.

Visualisation can be used to overcome any illness and can also be used to achieve whatever you want to achieve in your life. By creating a visual image or goal, you are making it happen by believing that it is possible. You then automatically remove any blocks preventing it from happening.

SILENT MEDITATION

Because our lives are so busy and full of activity, we seldom take time to balance this activity with a period of inactivity. This balance is essential for the proper functioning of the neuro-endocrine system and therefore of the whole body. Sleep is not necessarily a period of mental or emotional or indeed physical inactivity; your mind and emotions try to process what has happened during the day. Hence, your mind and emotions are often extremely active and some people can be quite physically active as well. Silent meditation is the way to balance the neuro-endocrine system. This is the key to healing the body. Through silent meditation we are able to withdraw from our busy lives, and through this withdrawal we can begin to gain insights into ourselves and how we are living our lives. This gives us more control over our lives and gives us the chance to implement necessary changes. Silent meditation is the single most important form of healing available to everyone, irrespective of religion, background, race or colour. Practise meditation for a minimum of thirty minutes daily and if possible involve the rest of your family.

Summary

In this chapter I have outlined the treatment of some of the more common digestive complaints. This has included mouth ulcers, halitosis, peptic ulcers, gallstones, irritable bowel syndrome, diverticulitis, constipation, inflammatory bowel disease (Crohn's disease and ulcerative colitis) and colon cancer. I have attempted to show what is available in natural medicine to assist these conditions.

I have not outlined the two most important digestive problems, i.e. dysbiosis and fermentation, both of which I have dealt with elsewhere in this book.

The single most important treatment modality is diet, regardless of the complaint.

The single most important nutrient to assist healing of the digestive tract is L-glutamine, an amino acid. Because it is an amino acid it is best taken between meals and in large quantities — two grams three times daily.

8

CONCLUSION: MAKING SENSE OF IT ALL!

In this book I have tried to give you a good general understanding of the most common digestive disorders that I have seen over the last fifteen years of practice. I have not dealt with digestive problems in children, as these are worthy of a separate book; I have stuck to adults only.

The truth is that almost any complaint that a patient presents with should be viewed as part of a digestive complaint until proven otherwise; that is how common digestive problems are, and that is how commonly they present as non-digestive symptoms. There is an epidemic of digestive problems in the modern world, so it is important to check everyone. I now routinely do tests on all my patients, including urine, stool and in some cases rectal swabs, blood tests and X-rays if these are appropriate. I try to stay away from invasive investigations as much as possible, as urine and stool tests can provide sufficient information to diagnose and treat; in cases where it does not I refer people for further tests until I have a clear idea of what is at the root of the problem. Because most of the tests that I order are not expensive, it is a suitable form of medicine for people who do not want to pay for expensive tests or who simply cannot afford them. When you realise that the price you might have to pay for not being tested in this simple, inexpensive way could be very high (i.e. you may develop a life-threatening disorder such as bowel cancer), you will see the need for all of us to be tested in this way at least once a year. This is preventative medicine at its best. If you have not visited your local practitioner, do not delay; mark in your diary to have checks done on urine and stool (as I have outlined in Chapter 1) at the end of this month and then annually afterwards. Personally, I have extensive tests done around the time of my birthday, which is an easy way of remembering; that way I don't have to mark it in a diary.

Practise preventative medicine by having your urine and stool checked once a year.

Your doctor should check the urine for indican, check the chemistry of the urine and if necessary do a mannitol and lactulose test to check for leaky gut syndrome. These tests will inform your doctor if you have gut fermentation (the indican test), leaky gut (the mannitol/lactulose test), diabetes (glucose present with or without ketones), or bleeding in the urinary tract (blood present).

The stool should be checked for parasites, the most common being: *Giardia lamblia, Entamoeba histolytica, Cryptosporidium.*

Your doctor should ask the laboratory to do microscopy on the stool sample and to check the intestinal flora. The microscopy will indicate if there is blood or mucus in the stool. If the flora result is abnormal, then dysbiosis can be diagnosed; the severity of the dysbiosis can be quantified by the laboratory, which is very useful to monitor progress.

These urine and stool analyses should be carried out once a year. In cases where treatment for dysbiosis is not proving effective or where progress is too slow I recommend colonic irrigation.

I shall now describe this process in more detail.

COLONIC IRRIGATION
This is a procedure where a small pipe is inserted into the back passage or anus and warm water is passed into the

colon all the way round to the caecum. This water softens impacted faecal matter and, with the help of a trained therapist who massages the abdomen, clears it out of the colon. The outlet pipe that carries the contents of the colon away has a glass section so that the therapist can see what is coming out and can therefore diagnose what problems exist internally. For example, if there are lots of white threads, like bits of cotton wool, this is diagnostic of candidiasis. In this way, colonic irrigation is not only useful as a form of treatment; it helps in a diagnostic sense as well.

Colonic irrgiation is helpful for anyone, but is particularly helpful in chronic conditions such as dysbiosis, fermentation and constipation.

Cleaning out impacted faecal matter is not the only way in which it can be of assistance; it can also be used to instil herbs and probiotics into the colon. Because colonic irrigation removes much of the bacterial flora in the colon, it is necessary to use a probiotic supplement afterwards.

Colonic irrigation is helpful for anyone, but particularly where there is a chronic intestinal problem. It is both diagnostic and therapeutic.

FERMENTATION AND DYSBIOSIS

Chapter 2 dealt with fermentation, a condition where instead of digesting starch and sugars you use them to manufacture your own wine and beer, and later, if you get good at it, the hard stuff! No, I am just joking! Many of the symptoms of fermentation and dysbiosis overlap, not surprisingly, since the two conditions usually co-exist. You need to have an overgrowth of yeast to ferment carbohydrates. The classic symptoms of fermentation are bloating, wind, gurgling and belching, caused by the excess gas produced by the fermentation process; this process also produces a lot of heat. So people who suffer from this condition tend to be intoxicated with the alcohols and aldehydes produced, blown up with gases, and overheated.

INTESTINAL FERMENTATION

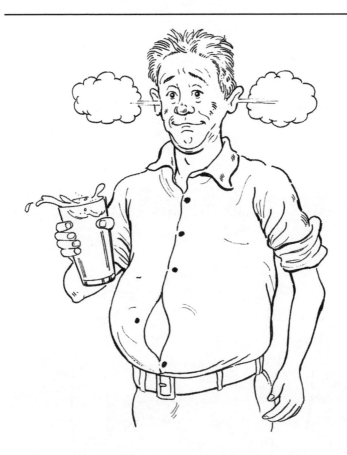

Fermentation is diagnosed by means of a urine test. Alcohol acts as a diuretic and so people with fermentation pass water more frequently; hence it is quite easy to get a urine sample from them. It can be diagnosed by testing the urine for indican. If this chemical is present it suggests that you are not digesting food properly.

The diet used to treat fermentation can initially be quite restrictive. Fasting can actually speed up the healing process if you feel so inclined; in fact, many people with this disorder often feel better when they eat little or nothing (although I

143

am not advocating that you eat nothing until you become skeletal in size in order to be cured!). In addition to diet it is necessary to support the digestive system and to treat the dysbiosis as well.

DYSBIOSIS

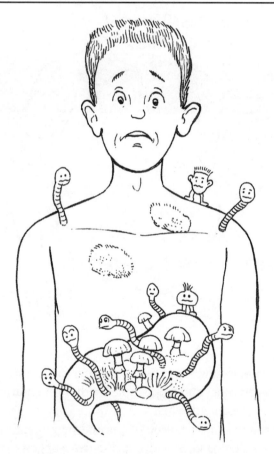

Dysbiosis often occurs on its own without fermentation. It is the single commonest condition in medical practice today. It is when 'gremlins' start to grow inside your intestines and slowly take over your body — pleasant thought, eh? Well, to put it a little less dramatically, it is when the 'baddies'

outnumber the 'goodies' and the 'baddies' start to gobble up some of your minerals and vitamins; not only that, they also demand sugar and yeast foods in ever-increasing quantities. In addition, there are not enough 'goodies' to manufacture many of the B vitamins that your body needs. So, to say that you end up being overwhelmed and invaded by parasites is really an understatement. However, the good news is that dysbiosis is eminently curable.

Dysbiosis is diagnosed by testing a stool sample. This is examined by laboratory technicians who can then inform your practitioner how many 'gremlins' you have growing inside you and in what quantities.

Treatment involves exterminating the enemy by: a) starving them, b) killing them with anti-microbials, and c) replacing them with good bacteria called probiotics. Some probiotic supplements contain extra food for the good bacteria; this extra food is called a prebiotic supplement and examples are inulin and fructo-oligosaccharide (FOS).

STRESS CAN HAVE A PROFOUND EFFECT ON DIGESTION

Prolonged stress causes shutdown. Saliva stops flowing, gastric juices dry up, deep breathing disappears, the pancreas slows down, digestion and absorption are disturbed, and elimination may be either excessive or non-existent. Stress underlies many digestive disorders, including dysbiosis, fermentation, leaky gut syndrome, peptic ulcers, irritable bowel syndrome. When stressed, instead of giving our bodies the extra help they need, we eat all the wrong foods, eat at the wrong times of day and we stop exercising. Having treated many hundreds of people over the years it seems that we love stress; in fact we're addicted to it — we humans are real adrenaline junkies, we just cannot get enough of it.

ADRENALINE JUNKIE

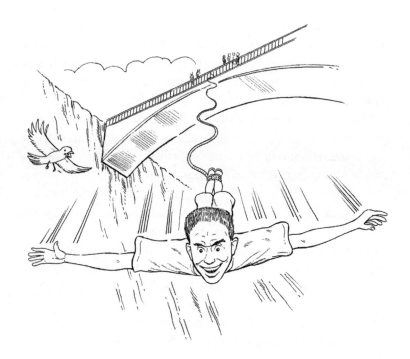

All junkies need counselling; all stress junkies need stress management as well.

Negative stress can disturb not only your digestion and respiration but your whole being. Seek help if you feel stressed and cannot cope with it.

EMOTIONS AND DIGESTION

How do our emotions affect our digestive systems and vice versa? It is true that our emotional state can exert a strong influence on the gut; digestive disorders can also exert a strong influence on our emotional well-being.

Many people with chronic digestive disorders tend to fall into one of two categories. Most of them have suppressed emotions such as anger; others tend to be highly sensitive people with wonderful gifts — healers, artists, musicians, etc., fall into this category. A person's emotional state alters the neuro-endocrine system in the gut, which tend in turn alters digestion, absorption and elimination as well as the immune system. Highly sensitive people have the ability to sense things that others cannot, but they are also much more sensitive to negativity, and there is no shortage of that in our modern world; they absorb this negativity like a sponge and then store it in their guts where it proceeds to wreak havoc. Negative emotions not only wreak havoc in our external world, but also disturb homeostasis in our internal world. Healing your emotional state and your coping mechanisms takes time; you also have to be ready to heal. Identifying that there is a problem is not sufficient; it has to cause you enough grief and pain that it drives you to seek help. As they say: 'no pain, no gain'. Healing or releasing suppressed emotions is a critically important process; if you don't do this, you will be forever going round in circles in your life until eventually you become consumed by the anger or fear or jealousy that you are carrying around with you. As I have mentioned in Chapter 5, these emotions affect every aspect of our being, but most especially the digestive system and, if left untreated, can end up causing life-threatening illnesses such as cancer. You must not get caught in a vicious cycle, with negative emotions leading to negative eating habits, leading to digestive problems, leading to more negative emotions and so on. Break out of the cycle and go for healing. Healthfood shops usually know everyone working in the field of alternative medicine and also know their reputations. In Ireland, there is a book called *Sláinte* which has a directory of who's who in the world of alternative medicine. Ring any practitioner in your area and find out what is happening. Healing brings the magic back into life and frees you to live like a child again, full of wonder and joy at being alive.

Heal any negative emotions that you might harbour inside you, especially if you have a chronic digestive problem.

SECONDARY EFFECTS

Digestive problems can affect many other parts of the body. This is probably the most important point in the whole book. Too many people fail to link a symptom in some other part of the body with a digestive disorder. I have learned this lesson the hard way. If a symptom or symptoms keep recurring, then the problem lies elsewhere and nine times out of ten it lies in the digestive tract. That's because the digestive tract is potentially the most toxic part of the body, and when these toxins enter the bloodstream the effects can be felt almost anywhere. The liver and kidneys are usually the first to feel the effects, then the brain, muscles and skin, as they have such a rich blood supply. Then other organs such as the reproductive system, joints, etc., can be affected also. Digestive disorders have long tentacles and can reach any part of the body — even your mental and emotional health can be affected. Remember that the digestive system can be quite silent even when in great difficulty and so it is often the secondary symptoms that a person will present with. Health spas across the world make people feel good by focusing virtually all their attention on digestive health. Fortunately, it is never too late. The potential for the digestive system, and the liver especially, to heal is enormous. If you want to halt the ageing process, i.e. the flabby skin, wrinkles on the face, age spots, aches and pains, etc., treat the digestive tract. Do not take digestion for granted. Be vigilant about everything you eat, check that you are digesting and absorbing properly, clean the colon regularly and use lots of probiotics, even if you do not have a digestive problem. Fasting for three days once a month and for two weeks once a year will help you in many ways.

Digestive health is the key to good mental, emotional and physical health. Digestive health is the key to retarding the ageing process.

HEALING A DIGESTIVE DISORDER

Treatment of digestive disorders using natural medicine is not complicated, but it can take time. There is no quick fix for a complex structure such as the small intestine, which is approximately 30 feet in length. You must exercise patience and expect lots of ups and downs. The graph in Figure 8.1 illustrates the difference between how people think they get better and how they actually get better.

The first important point to understand about healing a digestive disorder is that the function of the digestive tract is under the control of the involuntary nervous system, i.e. the adrenaline/non-adrenaline system. If you want to improve digestion then rest after eating and allow your digestive system to function efficiently. Also, because many of us are very busy during the day, it is very helpful to practise silent meditation for at least thirty minutes daily and teach your children to do this. All action and no rest makes Jack a dull and digestively disturbed boy!

Diet is the second important point regarding treatment of common digestive complaints. The gut will not heal until you ease its workload and remove any foods that may be upsetting it. If you have dysbiosis there is no good using pro-biotics and anti-microbials unless you cut out foods that aggravate the condition. I have tried to outline the correct diet for each digestive condition but if in doubt consult your practitioner.

The single most important food to consume daily is lots of purified water. The cells of your body are mostly water, so take a bottle of water with you as you go about your daily duties.

If you are not digesting food well then it is of prime importance to use digestive enzymes; there are many brands on the market and a healthfood shop attendant or your practitioner will help you choose one that is suitable for you.

Figure 8.1 *GETTING BETTER*

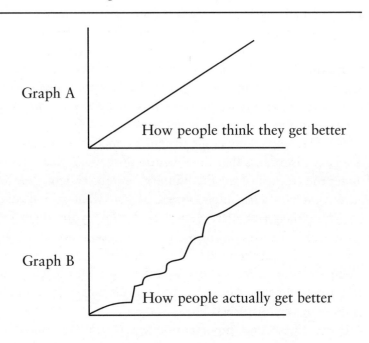

Getting better has ups and downs

The single most important nutrient to assist the healing of the digestive tract is L-glutamine, because it is the main nutrient for the cells that make up the gut lining.

Probiotics are also very important, as they constitute the best preventative medicine supplement available. People who have healthy intestinal flora are less likely to get serious intestinal problems such as bowel cancer. Use a probiotic supplement every day of your life; try to get one that has a prebiotic added to it, such as fructo-oligosaccharide or inulin; this will ensure the survival of the good bacteria as they travel along the digestive tract. Better still, when you are having colonic irrigation ask the therapist to instil some good bacteria into the colon afterwards. Two suppliers of probiotics are Higher Nature and Solgar, both based in the UK (see Appendix).

Cleaning the colon on a regular basis is another essential. This can be done using medicines or by colonic irrigation or by the use of enemas. A clean colon is a healthy colon. Do not allow toxic waste to remain in the colon. Empty, empty, empty!

Linseed oil is a wonderful food supplement to use because it bulks the stool and so helps elimination, and it also supplies the body with omega three oils, which many people lack.

One excellent product which will assist with almost any type of digestive complaint is 'Digestol'. It contains L-glutamine in high dosage, psyllium (to help elimination), FOS (fructo-oligosaccharide) and quercetin (a powerful antioxidant), as well as a number of herbs that aid digestion and heal the digestive tract, helping the intestinal flora:

Milk thistle — strong detoxifying herb as shown in clinical studies

Slippery elm — soothing, anti-inflammatory and healing for the intestinal wall

Gentian — aids digestion, prevents fermentation

Liquorice — stimulates bloodflow to the intestinal lining; assists the absorption of other herbs

Digestol assists digestion, absorption and elimination and will promote healing of the intestinal wall. It is a product that I have been using for some time now and has brought great relief to many of my patients. If you would like to try it, it can be sourced through a company in the UK called Nutrihealth (see Appendix).

Vigorous exercise is essential for good health,   but do a form of exercise that you enjoy — some people love dancing or hiking or canoeing rather than jogging. The form of exercise is not important. Just do something that excites you and you will not even be aware that you are exercising. Exercise is particularly stimulating for the intestinal tract, so if you suffer from digestive problems, exercise more often and more vigorously.

I have outlined the specific treatment for the most common digestive disorders in Chapters 2, 3 and 7. If you would like more information consult the bibliography at the end of the book.

I wish you happy eating, and happy digestion. May you live a long and healthy life.

When being treated for a digestive disorder be patient and expect ups and downs.

Appendix

USEFUL NAMES AND ADDRESSES
1. Pure H$_2$O
    Unit 5
    Egham Business Village
    Crabtree Road
    Egham
    Surrey TW20 8RB
    Tel: (01784) 221 188
    Email: *enquiries@pureh2o.co.uk*
2. Nutrihealth.UK
    Downlands Farm
    Drayton Lane
    Merston
    Chichester PO20 6EL
    Tel: (01243) 775 992
    Email: *enquiries@nutri-health.co.uk*
    They supply a small range of excellent, all-natural, products, one of which is Digestol.
3. Higher Nature
    Burwash Common
    East Sussex TN19 7BR
    Tel: (01435) 882 880
    Email: *sales@higher-nature.co.uk*
    They supply an excellent range of natural supplements including probiotics.
4. Solgar Vitamins
    Aldbury
    Tring
    Herts HP23 5PT
    Tel: (01442) 890 355
    They supply a range of natural medicines as well as pro-biotics.

5. Association of Colon Hydrotherapists
   16 Drummond Ride
   Tring
   Herts HP23 5DE
   Tel: (01442) 825 632
   Contact: Richard Wheeler
   They provide a list of therapists in your area who practise colonic irrigation.
6. Parascope Laboratory
   Dept of Microbiology
   Chapel Allerton Hospital
   Chapeltown Road
   Leeds LS7 4SA
   Tel: (0113) 392 4657
   Website: *www.parascope.co.uk*
   They do stool tests for fungi, yeast, parasites.
7. Biolab
   Stone House
   9 Weymouth Street
   London W1W 6DB
   Tel: (0207) 636 5959
   Email: *info@biolab.co.uk*
   They do tests for fermentation and leaky gut, as well as a lot of conventional medical tests, such as liver function and kidney function.
8. Nelson's Pharmacy
   Dame Street
   Dublin 2
   They supply homeopathic medicines.

BIBLIOGRAPHY

Ballantine, Rudolph, *Diet and Nutrition*, Honesdale, Pennsylvania: Himalayan Institute 1978.

Borysenko, Joan, *Minding the Body, Mending the Mind*, New York: Bantam Books 1987.

Chopra, Deepak, *Perfect Digestion*, New York: Harmony Books 1995.

Crook, William, *The Yeast Connection*, Jackson, Tennessee: Professional Books 1985.

Daniel, Rosy, *The Cancer Prevention Book*, London: Simon & Schuster 2001.

De Vries, Jan, *Stomach and Bowel Disorders*, Edinburgh: Mainstream Publishing 1994.

Garrett, Laurie, *The Coming Plague*, New York: Farrar, Straus & Giroux 1994.

Gawain, Shakti, *Creative Visualisation*, San Rafael, California: New World Library 1979.

Gittleman, Ann Louise, *Guess What Came to Dinner? Parasites & Your Health*, Garden City Park, New York: Avery Publishing 1993.

Janowitz, Henry, *Your Gut Feelings*, New York: Oxford University Press 1994.

Jonsson, Gudrun, *Gut Reaction*, London: Vermilion 1998.

Lipski, Elizabeth, *Digestive Wellness*, Lincolnwood, Illinois: Keats Publishing 2000.

McKenna, John, *Alternatives to Antibiotics*, Dublin: Newleaf 1996.

McKenna, John, *Alternatives to Tranquillisers*, Dublin: Newleaf 1999.

Murray, Michael and Joseph Pizzorno (eds), *The Encyclopaedia of Natural Medicine*, Rocklin, California: Prima Publishing 1991.

Oppenheim, Michael, *The Complete Book of Better Digestion*, Emmaus, Pennsylvania: Rodale Press 1990.

Peiken, Steven, *Gastrointestinal Health*, New York: HarperCollins 1991.

Randolph, Theron and Ralph Moss, *An Alternative Approach to Allergies*, New York: Harper & Row 1989.

Shabert, Judith and Nancy Erlich, *The Ultimate Nutrient: Glutamine*, Garden City Park, New York: Avery Publishing 1994.

Simonton, Carl and Stephanie Simonton, *Getting Well Again*, London: Bantam 1978.

Trenev, Natasha, *Probiotics: Nature's Internal Healers*, Garden City Park, New York: Avery Publishing 1999.

White, Erica, *Beat Candida Cookbook*, London: Thorsons 1999.

Whiteside, Mike, *Digestive Disorders*, London: Bloomsbury Publishing 1995.

INDEX